Dynamics of Yoga

...for Mubina with
Om & prem
Sascha
van
Yoga Sadhana

With kind regards, ॐ and prem

Swami Niranjan

Dynamics of Yoga

The Foundations of Bihar Yoga

Swami Satyananda Saraswati

Yoga Publications Trust, Munger, Bihar, India

Printed by Bihar School of Yoga
First published 1966
Reprinted 1973, 1976, 1983, 1997

Printed by Yoga Publications Trust
Second edition 2002
Reprinted 2006, 2007

ISBN: 81-85787-14-X

Publisher and distributor: Yoga Publications Trust, Ganga Darshan, Munger, Bihar, India.

Website: www.yogavision.net

Printed at Thomson Press (India) Limited, New Delhi, 110001

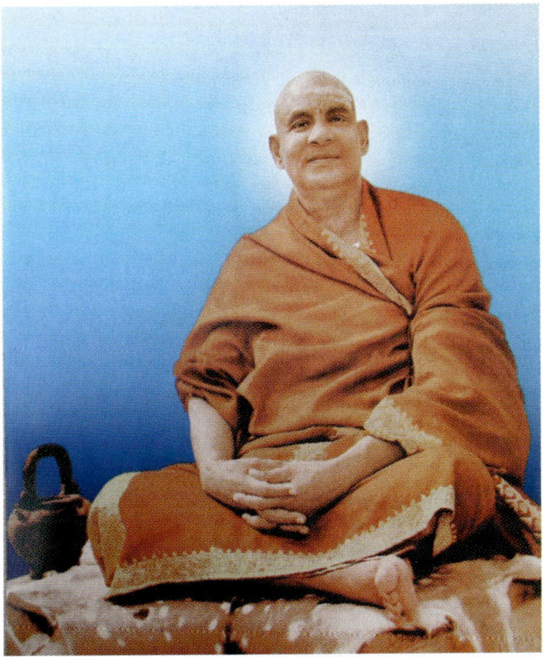

Dedication

In humility we offer this dedication to
Swami Sivananda Saraswati, who initiated
Swami Satyananda Saraswati into the secrets of yoga.

Contents

Introduction

There are many books on yoga. Some have been written by yogis from India, and have dealt mostly with the more abstract aspects of yoga like dhyana and samadhi. Other books have been written by authors from western countries, who have tended to emphasize the more tangible, physical potentialities of applied yoga, such as asana and pranayama. However, the vast potential of psycho-physiological therapy; its unlimited scope on the spiritual path; its unequalled utility as a way of life which leads to happiness in the trying circumstances of the fast-changing, modern world; and its bright future as the culture of tomorrow – these aspects of yoga have not yet been explained in detail.

Many people associate yoga with hermits sitting on mountain peaks or in caves, with people who sleep on beds of nails or do strange things in general. Most people in the world, however, have no concept about yoga at all, for little has been done to explain yoga in terms that they can easily understand, devoid of the trappings of esoteric 'mumbo-jumbo'. It is hoped that this book will help people to understand yoga and to realize that it is a science very much concerned with modern living.

We believe that a systematic effort, in the form of a movement to propagate yoga in its broadest sense on an international basis, will tear asunder the veil of mystery surrounding yoga and that yoga will eventually emerge in all its pristine glory and truth. Yoga is not for a select few individuals, but is for all the young and the old, the fit and the ailing, the rich and the poor. With its infinite resources and potential it will usher mankind into a new and glorious era of evolution.

This book is but a small token of our dedication to the cause of yoga and an attempt to explain yoga and yogic techniques in a clear and unambiguous language. It is a humble offering.

Yoga Explained

New Horizons of Yoga

Laymen have very vague and often strange ideas on yoga. But even those who have some knowledge of this ancient science and have come into practical contact with it, often find it difficult to appreciate some of its more obvious truths. Indeed, a few of the ideas propounded in this chapter may appear to be new and will very likely uproot many pet theories on yoga.

What are these new ideas? Firstly, it is not essential to leave one's house or go into oblivion to practise yoga. It is time we discarded the belief that only renunciates or monks (*sannyasins*) are fit to practise yoga. Secondly, marital relations do not present any obstacle in the practice of yoga. Thirdly, non-vegetarians need not give up their food habits just because they have taken to yoga. The real aim of yoga is to attain peace and tranquility within. For attaining this, you need not give up any of your normal ways of living.

Running away from the difficulties of life is not the way to deliverance. The battlefield of life is not illusory. It may be illusory to the philosopher; his world is one of imagination and his feet are not firmly planted on the ground. Yoga is practical and has nothing to do with philosophical flights of fancy. Never believe for a moment that a householder's station in life is inferior and that a renunciate's or monk's station in life is superior, and let no woman think that her status in life is inferior to that of a man.

Yoga has a special role to play in the world of today. Its practice alone can remove mental and physical afflictions. It can bring joy into our hearths and homes. Yoga does not lay down extraordinary conditions of self-discipline and behaviour patterns. You can continue enjoying the good things of life and still be a yogi; nor is it at all necessary to give up the worldly ambitions or material aspirations to take to the yogic way of life. However, one need not become a slave of one's desires.

Those who sincerely practise yoga remain undisturbed, like an ocean which receives the turbulent waters of inrushing rivers. While enjoying sense-gratifications a yogi is careful not to allow them to overpower him. It does not help to despise life. There is no virtue in retiring to the woods and sitting enchanted in the solitary grandeur of *samadhi* (super-conscious state of self-equilibrium). Heroism lies in remaining steadfast in the tumult of life even when the scales are heavily loaded against us, and in attaining the samadhi of equilibrium in the midst of all odds.

A physician who wants only healthy persons for his patients is no physician. Likewise, if yoga were to work its wonders only on the physically and mentally fit, it would cease to be an amazing science of life; its scope would be very much limited. Being a highly rational science, yoga can benefit all people under all circumstances of life. After the daily round of mental and physical toil it can bring back resilience and vigour and restore equipoise.

For worldly people life is a continuous sacrifice. Their labours to keep the home fires burning, their activities to discharge social, national and international responsibilities are oblations. Once this truth is understood, the vision of self-realization can be kept undimmed even in the midst of unremitting hard work enjoined by one's station in life.

Ceaseless activity in the turmoil of life takes its own toll. Anxieties, frustrations, exhaustion of mind and body – all these accelerate the ageing process. Yoga is a powerful remedy against these forces of destruction.

Is life-long celibacy an indispensable condition, notwithstanding what the wise yogis of old have declared, for the pursuit of the soul-lifting science of yoga? The answer is no. Age also is no barrier. Whether one is on the threshold of life, or in the spring of youthfulness or has yielded to the venerableness of old age – anyone can learn yoga. In yoga there are no limiting factors.

Yoga does not mean solely the *ashtanga yoga* (yoga of the eight-fold path) described in the Hindu scriptures. Simple practices such as a regular course of *asana* (yogic postures), *pranayama* (yogic breathing practices), *japa* (repetition of mantra), *nada yoga* (yoga of sound vibration) and *trataka* (yogic gazing, akin to crystal gazing) are also very effective. *Karma yoga* (yoga of action), *bhakti yoga* (yoga of devotion), *jnana yoga* (yoga of enquiry) and *raja yoga* (yoga of meditation) are all different facets of yoga. Music being an integral part of it, bhakti yoga has a soothing effect on the bottled-up emotions and a fevered mind. Why go that far? Life itself is yoga. Our day-to-day work is yoga. The field is vast and inviting. Let the thrill and quiver of yoga transform all our activities in life.

In the snares and pitfalls of life, one cannot allow oneself to be divorced from reality. Patanjali's *yamas* (moral abstinences) and *niyamas* (observances of conduct of character), as popularly interpreted, were for an age that is gone and done with. The simple adamantine fact is that they have no place, if professed according to these interpretations, in the world of today. In the good old days the air that our ancestors breathed was full of these virtues. The vitiated air that we breathe today is full of falsehoods, violence and countless other imperfections. Truth (*satya*), non-injury (*ahimsa*), etc., are admittedly forces of great potency, but they are so only if one practises them to perfection in obedience to an inner compulsion. Yoga is not concerned with the cultivation of impossible virtues. We had better leave them to the moralist. Yoga is a rational science with technical systems for stilling the turbulent mind, for harnessing the physical and mental energies and for maintaining resilience. In a word, yoga aims at developing an integrated personality. The best way to achieve this is a synthesis of bhakti, karma, jnana and raja yogas. Man should not be all intellect, he should not be all emotion. There should be a happy blend of both, otherwise, there will be no peace in his life.

The word yoga is of great significance. It is derived from the Sanskrit root *yuj* (unite). Yoga means union, identification. Identify with the joys and sorrows of everyone, extend your horizons, live above the pettiness of life. If you take yoga in this sense, it ceases to be individualistic. Just as a mother and child have emotional identification, so should you have an emotional integration with all around you.

Yoga stands for both physical and mental well-being. It comes to suffering humanity as a blessing in the guise of psychosomatic treatment. It comes to the seekers of truth as the shortest way to God-realization. Indeed, yoga is a blueprint of perfection. You can consider it as a program, a method and a philosophy. It is a program, insofar as it assumes the shape of a movement with definite aims and objects. It is a method in the sense that yogic practices are methodically pure. Whatever may be one's spiritual orientation, meditation and other practices can always be very useful. Few methods of self-realization are so universally valid and practicable. Thus, yoga is a universal recipe and is truly the only modus operandi for self-realization.

People make very noble resolves; they want self-realization, they wish to follow high ideals. But there is a snag – they have no willpower. There can be no material or spiritual progress without willpower. Do not develop a split personality: a show of willpower in public but pandering to weakness in secrecy – a conflict between ego and super-ego.

Do you enjoy a happy, harmonious life? Are you afire with enthusiasm in your daily activities? When adverse circumstances try to crush you, do you rise above them with a cool head and easy assurance? If not, take to yoga.

Yoga and Physical Hygiene

The psycho-physiological aspect of yoga is of profound importance. This ancient science never regards man as a mere biological entity. The ancient thinkers paid great attention to the functioning of the mind and the inner mechanism. Today, psychology has also accepted this basic aspect in its scope of investigation and is increasingly recognizing the correlation between the body and the mind.

It thus becomes patent that for the progress of man in any field of activity, it is necessary that he should possess not only a healthy body but also a healthy mind. Yoga has always aimed at the emergence of a healthy and integrated personality in man as the indispensable condition for his ability to take to higher flights in yoga. No wonder, therefore, that Patanjali has reaffirmed the technique of ashtanga yoga in both its aspects – technically known as *bahiranga* (external) and *antaranga* (internal) – for the perfection of yoga. Those that fall into the first category are yama, niyama, asana and pranayama. Those classed in the second category are *pratyahara* (withdrawal or control of the senses), *dharana* (concentration), *dhyana* (meditation) and *samadhi* (superconscious state of self-equilibrium).

The first four constitute the fundamentals of physical hygiene. Yama, niyama, asana and pranayama are the cornerstones of physical hygiene for all. Then again, hatha yoga prescribes six purificatory techniques, the *shatkarmas* viz. *neti* (nasal cleaning), *dhauti* (internal cleansing), *basti* (yogic enema), *nauli* (abdominal massaging), *trataka* and *kapalbhati* (purification of the cranial region). All these constitute important techniques of physical hygiene. The ancient science of yoga fully realizes that the spinal cord and the brain constitute the central nervous system, and therefore strives to keep them in a healthy condition. In yoga, the proper functioning of the endocrine glands and the chemical reactions in the body are considered important. The aspirant, therefore, cheerfully subjects himself to a voluntary moderation in life, not necessarily denying the basic necessities of life (nor even resorting to suppressions of his instinctual urges) but by making a steady and assiduous effort in always trying to transmute these urges towards a higher purpose.

Therefore, asana, *mudra* (balancing exercises and inner attitudes) and pranayama are the main techniques which are followed to keep the physical system fit and healthy. These form the main supports for health, for yoga requires long and steady practice in one sitting posture.

Asanas are postures; they are not merely physical exercises that affect the muscular system. In yoga, muscular strength has not much importance and the body is only an instrument.

Fatigue, exhaustion, sloth, etc. are avoided in yoga practice. The attempt is always to keep the mind cheerful. The asanas constitute a technique which, when practised daily, re-tones and revitalizes the whole human system.

The central nervous system is the reservoir of all energy. There are latent centres in the body that are inactive and need to be activated. Asanas can help with this to some extent. Though said to be eighty-four in number, the principal asanas are few. Backward bending postures like *bhujangasana* (cobra pose), *shalabhasana* (locust pose) and *dhanurasana* (bow pose); forward bending postures like *halasana* (plough pose) and *paschimottanasana* (back stretching pose); twisting postures like *ardha matsyendrasana* (half spinal twist pose); inverted postures like *sarvangasana* (shoulder stand pose), *sirshasana* (head stand) – all keep the spinal column supple. According to yoga anatomy, the principal *nadi* (pranic channel), *sushumna,* passes through the spinal column. Of the fourteen principal nadis, the main three are *ida, pingala* and *sushumna.* The asanas keep the spinal column supple and toned up to enable the seeker to release his energy through the psychic passage within it.

The shatkarmas referred to above merely help in keeping the internal organs clean. The central nervous system alone is not of importance. The body also has endocrine glands: the pineal, pituitary, thyroid, parathyroid, thymus, etc. These glands secrete hormones and their secretions flow into the bloodstream. It is, therefore, essential to keep these functioning properly as they not only contribute to the development of the physical organism, but also influence the personality structure in a subtle way. Yoga thus enters the field of physiological-psychology. The mudras are natural exercises aiming at revitalization of the glands and the internal organs. These are *yoga mudra, maha mudra, maha bheda mudra* and so on. The mudras are also essential yogic techniques for physical health.

The third important technique is that of pranayama. It has a two-sided effect. It helps to keep the physical apparatus pure and in good order, and also to control, regulate and channel the mental-emotional being of man. Pranayama means controlled, rhythmical and regular breathing. *Prana* is the gross manifestation in the physical body of the subtle, universal, cosmic force. It is this cosmic energy that gives life to all sentient beings. Pranayama is the technique of conservation and distribution of this life force.

While inhaling the respiratory system takes in oxygen, and while exhaling it discharges carbon dioxide. Oxygenation of the system makes the body pure, light and active. Unless the science of breathing is properly understood and correctly practised, there is a likelihood of imbalance in breathing, which may result in various types of mental and emotional conflicts and impulsiveness. The world with its innumerable joys and sorrows makes a violent impact upon us and we often fail to find a realistic adjustment to life. The effect of prana on the human being and the correlation between the mind and the body are fully realized in yoga.

Thus yoga has a substantial contribution to make to, and a scientific and potent part to play in, the field of physical hygiene.

Yoga and the Mind

The mind is the most mysterious component of the body. It is the cause of both pleasure and pain. Even with this knowledge, philosophers and seers have failed to harness it. The mind is that agent which receives and disposes of all knowledge and controls physical activities. It functions in various capacities. Automatic reflex action and thoughtful deliberations are both actuated by mental waves. The proper functioning of the mind cannot be grasped unless we take account of neurological and phrenological researches.

The ancient science of yoga as enunciated by *rishis* of old relates to us the process of harnessing the mind. Schopenhauer once wrote that desires are infinite and fulfilment is limited. Will has more power to grasp than attain. The best way to ensure happiness is to have minimum wants and desires. One desire leads to another associated desire and the process goes on endlessly. This is true. The eastern philosophers and saints have been telling us for ages that the mind is the cause of happiness and sorrow. One who conquers the mind goes beyond the reach of pain and pleasure.

But how to conquer the mind? We believe it can be achieved through yoga alone. Peace or liberation is nowhere beyond this earth and it is to be acquired here and now by the proper mental discipline. In the *Bhagavad Gita*, which is an unparalleled document on yoga, Lord Krishna said to

Arjuna: "Merge your mind and intellect in Me and there is no doubt that you will be one with Me." Thus, the Lord has asked us to merge the mental personality with the divine.

In order to realize the supreme self, the vagaries of the mind are to be checked. The mind should be perfectly calm and unruffled. Then alone, during the hours of deep concentration and contemplation, does the light of the soul dawn on us. In simple words, dhyana – meditation and contemplation – is the only way to realize the self or superconscious perception.

To practise dhyana, i.e. to harness the mind, is a difficult job. Yet constant practise and a resolute will is the surest way to success. You cannot expect meditation to be perfected in a day or two. An aspirant should never feel disheartened at his failures; he should go on with his meditation relentlessly till the goal is reached.

Meditation, perfect or imperfect, is essential for all. Why? The mind is like a pond of water and even a little breeze of thought can disturb its surface. Constant thought waves create tensions which bring on ageing, which in turn ebbs away the strength in a short time. Man is not a mere bottle of blood, a mass of flesh and a bundle of bones; he is full of likes and dislikes, ideals, faith and feelings. From the cradle to the grave he goes on filling his basket of life with agreeable experiences. His mind thus becomes very much a lumber room of sensations, perceptions and conceptions. All these overpower his divine nature.

Had these experiences been of one life only, it would have been easy to wipe out the impressions of the mind and make it a *tabula rasa* (clean slate) again. But man is reborn to work out the actions of his past lives. He comes with a rich store of *anadi vasana* (beginningless instincts) which may be called impressions and experiences of many lives. All these block his supreme awareness and it is his task in the new life given to him, to wipe them out.

An aspirant has, therefore, to deal with his present as well as his immediate and distant past. An aspirant is he who has traversed the indulgent way of life where his attention was only on gaining sense experience, but realizing that desires have no end, he wishes now to set his foot on withdrawal, leaving them all behind.

Raja yoga is a branch of yoga which devises the techniques of dhyana (meditation) for physical, mental and spiritual unfoldment. Meditation is a process of exhausting the hidden, latent and suppressed desires of the unconscious. Man has in him suppressed emotions too. If these suppressed emotions and desires are not rooted out, they will manifest themselves in the form of personality errors, physical and mental illnesses like neuroses, psychoses, nervous breakdowns and high blood pressure, etc. A man who has mastered his emotions and feelings, and risen above petty desires, can never get ill unless it is time to leave his mortal abode.

Meditation for a few minutes is a tonic for everyone. The mind feels relaxed during concentration. During meditation, persistent efforts made to bring the mind back (time and again) to one and the same object save the energies of the mind from being wasted. Instead of shifting from one thought to another and generating waves of different frequencies, it begins to revolve round one object, generating waves of one and the same frequency. This practice of meditation economizes mental energies. It calms and controls the astral body. Rhythmic vibrations are generated, soothing both the body and the mind. Meditation restores the vitality of the mind. It makes up the loss caused by aimless and useless brooding and painful thoughts of the day.

Thus, meditation helps to wipe out past experiences and at the same time avoids accumulation of new ones. It serves as a useful and sound strategy to guard against unpleasant shocks which we receive in the world. Life is a struggle which is to be won by strengthening the mind as well as the body. Yoga is a burning furnace which gives a new pattern to body and mind and makes them strong enough to face the tempests and tumults of the world.

Everyone has to come out of life with courage and fortitude. Yoga offers sure techniques of controlling the mind, to equip oneself with courage and certitude to face life squarely and to work out one's final emancipation.

It is well-known that mind and body act and react on each other. Mental ailments cause physical ailments and vice versa. We allow our senses to run hither and thither to hunt for physical satiety. We identify ourselves too much with the body, which results in neurosis and frustrations. Yoga offers a remedy for the reconstruction of our personality: withdraw the senses from their objects and go within the 'middle chamber', the subconscious of the psychologists. When we contact our subconscious through meditation, one after another, all our deep-rooted past impressions come to the surface and slowly but surely depart from us. This process is entirely in accord with modern psychiatric practices, with the difference, however, that here we are our own psychiatrists.

Modern civilization has made man abnormal. He is sick physically and mentally. He hugs pain and broods over melancholy thoughts. Medicines may soothe temporarily but offer no cure. By deep meditation alone can we overcome mental, physical and emotional tensions and rid the world of its besetting maladies.

Objectives of Meditation

Meditation is a way to self-realization. If you sit down for it you will find it very difficult. Many problems will come forward. How to meditate may be your first problem. Even interested seekers are generally quite ignorant of the techniques of meditation. It is not easy to forget body consciousness and to force the mind to dwell for long on a single desired object. Mastery over the mind cannot be achieved in one day. No school can give you a certificate of qualification on the very first day of admission. It takes a long time to score anything in the field of meditation. Meditation is a very vague term giving no idea of its program to the new aspirant.

Meditation is an exercise in mental discipline. It disciplines and directs the mind towards a desired end. It is the subjective approach to disciplining the mind. It is a way to control the vagaries of the mind. People suffering from inner conflicts due to divergent emotions, such as worry, anxiety, indecisiveness etc., are greatly benefited by the practice of meditation. It gives a chance for introspection and clears the maladies of the inner self. The twentieth-century man remains extrovert the whole day. He finds little time to look within, which is most essential. Even the busiest man has to find time to nurse his physical body. In the same manner your inner self also requires a few minutes attention daily. If the physical body needs evacuation, a wash, a refill and garments to wear, will your mental body not need something of an abstract nature? Your mind without a moment's rest is facing the stress and strain of life. Therefore, it needs careful tending. Even machines are put to rest after a certain number of hours work. Can you name a single technique to remove and ease the tensions of the nerves except the yogic methods of relaxation and revitalization? The accumulation of thought-wastes can be brushed away by no other method than the process of meditation.

Diseases or functional disorders of the nervous system like neurosis, neurasthenia, etc. can be successfully treated by meditation. Applied meditation has a great deal to contribute to medical therapy. Meditational therapy will cure psychoneuroses – the various illnesses that arise in people who are in no sense insane. Meditation is also useful in the prevention, as well as cure, of several diseases. Cases of psychoses can also be successfully treated.

Meditation awakens the inner self. Through meditation the latent or unused faculties of the mind or the brain centres are awakened. If the mind is set free from memories of past experiences even for the time being – if it is absolutely tensionless and one-pointed – its energies can be directed towards the exploration of the unknown, unseen and unheard regions. Some transcendental knowledge dawns through the thin cut made by the pointed mind. Should the mind take up a problem and work upon it for several hours, days, months, or years, it sees a new light, discovers a new approach, and finds a solution to the problem. This is what great scientists have realized. Deep, concentrated, one-pointed meditation opens a new vista of life or knowledge.

All the vicissitudes of mind are yet unknown to mankind. The greatest of the scientists admit that the ultimate truth is not yet known. Meditation may assist in rooting out several diseases like blood pressure, pain, etc. Its therapeutic efficacy has already been discussed.

The great psychologist, Sigmund Freud, maintained that the occurrences on the physical plane are but manifestations of unconscious desires. If this is true, the root of all misery, ailment and illness is the blessed id of Freud. The Hindu psychologists of old have also maintained similar views, but for the difference in terminology. Freud's id is nothing but a glimpse of *chitta*, the storehouse of all desires and primitive instincts. All diseases originate in the mind first. The mere idea or fear that 'I may catch cold' or 'I may contract a disease' prepares the body for reception of the germs. The regular practice of meditation develops the willpower and frees the mind from the arrest of wrong notions, whims and fears.

An argument may be advanced, for example, that a child, whose thinking is not mature, contracts disease. Why? Experiments have shown that a child is merely a psychological being. A child of tender age has developed the sense of taste, receptivity to surroundings, environment and atmosphere, etc. It is a different thing whether the child has learnt the art of expression or not. The child experiences, but lacks expression. Close observation of a child's behaviour has proved that a child is more sensitive than his elders. Children instinctively recognize love, anger, hatred, etc. They contract diseases because their minds and bodies are both in infancy. After attaining physical and mental maturity they will learn to resist the germs mentally.

Meditation leads to samadhi, the culmination of the evolution of the human mind. Through concentration, contemplation and meditation, one transcends the limits of mind. The mind and body are the two thorns that prick the soul of man and cause pain and misery. If the mind and body are both extinct, there can be no pain, no suffering, no sorrow, no ignorance, and nothing may bind or limit the power of the soul. A bird freed from the cage can soar to any height. Likewise, when consciousness, or the self or the soul, transcends the limits of mind and body, it enjoys supreme bliss, supreme power, supreme light. It may be wrong to say it enjoys. To be more correct, there will be no duality – no dual existence of consciousness, of knower and known. Consciousness becomes one, a part of the supreme consciousness or the cosmic consciousness.

If, through the instrument of non-attachment to external objects or desires, you sincerely practise and succeed in turning your mind towards transcendental objects, it will give up its age-long habit of reacting to the trifling incidents of life.

Samadhi: The Culmination of Yogic Effort

Trance, ecstasy, or suspension of consciousness is not samadhi. Samadhi is sublime equanimity. There are many wrong notions about samadhi. According to some, samadhi is a state in which one's body becomes like stone, the pulse rate slows down and the metabolic process stops. Suspended animation is a great science mastered by some yogis, but this is not samadhi. In the state of suspended animation there is no awareness or knowledge. The stock of subconscious elements, or the subliminal stock, remains unexhausted and dormant.

If samadhi merely meant a stage of steady posture and total unconsciousness, very few spiritual seekers would be successful in attaining it. A person who has been able to make the conscious and subconscious forces dormant deserves commendation but this has nothing to do with yoga and the common man. If the attainment of samadhi does not exhaust the muscular, emotional and other tension; if it does not bestow peace, power and enlightenment; if it does not remove your complexes, conflicts, schizophrenia and other such psychological disorders, it is certainly not samadhi.

What, then, is samadhi? Can everyone achieve samadhi? Is samadhi total awareness or complete forgetfulness? Is samadhi total suspension, forgetfulness, unconsciousness, inertia, or is it total awareness or absolute consciousness?

The mind is a bundle of mental patterns of awareness. When every pattern of awareness has been rejected and annihilated, what remains is the ultimate form of consciousness and it is here that man experiences peace within.

Modern man feels tension in his day-to-day life. The busy mechanical life of towns, the congestion due to industrial development, family problems – all these form the basis of his increased tension. Tension is that state in which two forces pull in opposite directions. When you want to do something in a particular manner, some force within dissuades you from doing so. This is tension, or conflict between ego and super-ego, as the psychoanalysts would describe it.

There are divine as well as evil elements in us. The war between the dark and the divine forces in us is the real tension. A psychologist will make you relax by certain methods, but then there is an inexhaustible stock of dormant subliminal and unsubliminal tendencies called *anadi vasana*. The psychologist cannot help you in exhausting this stock. It is here that yoga comes to our help. It has therapeutic, mental, spiritual, occult and psychic value.

If you wish to remove your tensions, firstly you have to ease and relax yourself. Find out the first, ultimate and original cause of tension. That tension is the constant struggle between the dark and the divine forces within us – between the devil and God. Through yoga, the mental, muscular and emotional tensions are removed and a stage dawns where there is an end to this eternal fight within. This is the supreme stage of sublime equanimity. Suspended animation has nothing to do with this. Yoga helps to make life powerful, to awaken the dormant genius within, to get insight and to activate the 'third eye' (the centre of intuition). This is the state of super-consciousness.

If you close your eyes, you will feel blankness and darkness within but in the yogic state of samadhi you are aware both internally and externally. This, however, is not the highest samadhi. The greatest samadhi is the balance of mind, not just the balance of consciousness. It is not the intellectual balance. Sometimes when you feel that there is no tension in you, the tension has actually passed on from the conscious level to the subconscious or the unconscious.

The greatest tension one feels when one advances in the stage of meditation is in his innermost body. The individual soul is in wilderness. The outgoing senses have taken away the peace of the individual soul. The individual soul comes into being out of intelligence, restlessness and inertia. Because of inertia the individual soul wanders in worldliness. The individual soul runs after shadows, greed, etc., and gives up the four factors necessary for peace. The company of holy persons, introspection, spiritual practice and inner silence are the four prongs of the way to set out in search of ultimate peace.

This is the point where the real tension starts. You have hitherto found pleasure in the world, developed hankering, craving and desire. Your fight is now with sloth, lethargy and indolence. You have also to fight with the unseen forces of mind, the conflicts in your consciousness. Devotion, spiritual vital strength, constant vigilance and ever-mindfulness are essential to progress. Your spiritual practice must be continuous and the tempo must be constant.

Sometimes even vigilance and mindfulness fail. Eclipsed by lethargy, vigilance is relaxed because the senses are very powerful. While fish, deer, elephants and serpents have only one sense active, which more often causes the loss of their life, man has five strong senses. Imagine the lot of a man who surrenders himself to his senses.

The individual has to take to spiritual practice in right earnest, without any postponement. If you postpone the program of your spiritual practice, it will never come in your life. Due to lack of constant vigilance and spiritual alertness the spiritual personality goes into oblivion. Therefore, always 'keep awake'. Lust, anger and greed are the great dacoits hidden in us and they loot our divine treasures. Therefore, be ever watchful.

How to get rid of the inner tensions? So long as you do not practise yoga, do not introvert your mind and control your senses, you will not be able to remove your tensions. The senses and mind are indestructible. Without craving there can be no mental activity. Craving or desire is the root cause of the war between the divine and the devil. So there is no use curbing the senses and suppressing the mind and sense desires. If you want spiritual peace, sublime equanimity, or the ultimate eternal peace, you will have to burn or annihilate attachment and perfect the art of detachment. There has to be no liking for pleasant things and no dislike for unpleasant things. Physical, mental or intellectual detachment will not help you much. Spiritual detachment is the real thing.

When the stock of anadi vasana is exhausted, there comes a state of perfect balance and peace. You will be what you are. You will be conscious of all things as you are conscious now. Samadhi is the state of absolute sense, intelligence and vigilance. You will recognize and know all in samadhi just as you know people in the waking state. You will maintain the normal sense of discrimination, but your mental, intellectual, political, social and sexual jaundice; your physical, mental and intra-intellectual crises will be overcome.

One does not become inactive after samadhi. Rather, one becomes very powerful and active. Hard work for days together does not tire. One does not need sleeping pills and tranquilizers. No incident of tragedy or joy has any influence. There is equipoise in joy and sorrow, death and birth, loss and gain, insult and praise, notoriety and fame. One is full of indescribable serenity. You must have experienced the serenity of deep sleep during which you are in the lap of a blissful experience and nothing disturbs you. The only difference between deep sleep and samadhi is that in sleep you are unconscious, while in samadhi you are conscious of everything and yet you are serene, equibalanced and cheerful. Imagine this highest state of bliss, peace and joy!

Every individual needs this attainment to face the storms of daily life with a balanced mind. You must have such strength that you do not get tired even after long working hours. If you take a rest, you must feel tired; if you eat, you must feel hunger; if you take medicine you must fall sick. Know the body, its laws, and the law-maker. It is possible to live without eating, sleeping, etc., but this is possible only after the attainment of samadhi, not before that.

Samadhi has been rightly regarded as a 'consummation devoutly to be wished for'. We do not consider samadhi as merely a practice. We must strive to attain perennial samadhi and personify it. Ours should be what is called an 'effortless and felicitous' samadhi.

Modern man has developed many scientific superstitions. You have to do away with them. Each and every idea finds currency with us without proper examination. Accept yoga in your daily life. Yoga is a way of life, the culture of tomorrow. It is not necessary that you should go to a temple or meditate on your deity; wherever you perceive, perceive with sublime equanimity.

For worldly achievements also you have to take to yoga. It will fulfil your worldly ambitions and quench your spiritual thirst. Whether you wish for good health, for happy marital life or prosperity or spiritual enlightenment, yoga will help you. The starting point of yoga is the company of holy persons and good books. Its culmination is in samadhi. You will always remain restless if you do not practise yoga. There will be something wrong with your inner personality. The first, last and the only remedy for the removal of emotional, muscular and mental tensions is the practice of yoga. It is only then that you will be free from all tensions and reach a stage where you will exclaim with joy and ecstasy – 'I am happy, I am happy, I am happy!'

Yoga Philosophy: A Preface

We are living in an exciting age, an age of constant revolution in the human realm. The sciences have ushered in a technological era and civilization has reached its materialistic apex, with a great revolution in human thinking also. The Freudian psychology, with its offshoot of the neo-Freudian group, has demonstrated new dimensions of human personality. In biology, physics, chemistry, astrology, astronomy, ethics, philosophy and psychology, new vistas of knowledge have been opened up.

A bird's-eye view of history demonstrates the fact that in every age man has felt that he is living in a unique age. It is, however, indisputable that the twentieth century brought progress to a point of no return. So, it is all the more necessary to consolidate and preserve the instruments and results of progress than to rush forward to achieve more than mankind could use profitably. A mental revolution should match the technological revolution in the right perspective and in good faith. It is here that a need for resurrection of ancient values is keenly felt. While facts change, values remain constant. So, what was fundamental to the concept of good life and harmonious progress is still fundamental and not vitiated by changes in the social, political and economic spheres. Truth, beauty and goodness are ideals which have received different interpretations, yet they endure as the ultimate pursuits of mankind.

Yoga, both in its philosophy and in its technique, is a means to the attainment of these ideals. Therefore, the paramount need of the day is to redeem yoga from oblivion and to restore it to its place of pride in the scheme of human knowledge.

The word yoga has been used, misused and abused. To some it is a relic of the past. To others, it has a host of scaring implications. Yoga is a popular word and also an ancient word. Much before Patanjali envisaged his philosophy of yoga, which was in fact an indirect systematization of Samkhya metaphysics, the term yoga had been referred to in several Hindu scriptures and also in Buddhist literature. The confusion has been confounded by the piecemeal approach to yogic theory. The emphasis on yogasanas (necessary though they are) to the exclusion of the philosophy and metaphysics of yoga has in the long run reduced yoga to a method of body-building. Today people also fight shy of the term yoga because of its unsavoury implication that to live a yogic life is to live an asocial life of seclusion and self-abnegation. Popular misconceptions about yoga are still rampant and some of them are too immature to be taken seriously. Nonetheless, this climate of misinterpretation has to be destroyed and a reassertion of yogic values has to be made.

Man, to repeat a platitude, is a philosophical animal. In fact, he is the only animal who has a hunger and thirst for perfection. The history of mankind shows that at every stage we have been trying to perfect our social, political and religious institutions so that we can live a life free from all ills, devoted to the study and realization of the Ultimate. Yoga philosophy is directed to this end, but its processes are prescribed at all levels of human personality. Yogic philosophy realizes that body, as the abode of soul, is as important as mind; that physiology demands equal attention to psychology. Beginning with bodily discipline, the yoga system goes on to the transformation of the mental set-up by prescribing several different kinds of exertions of mind.

It is only after integration between a sound body and vigorous mind that a sublime synthesis between the individual soul and the universal soul can be attained.

On the level of the body, no extra thought or expenditure of mental energy is required to demonstrate that good health can be kept up by good discipline. It is no self-abnegation to deny yourself that food which upsets your stomach. It is no sacrifice to desist from those delicacies which make one ill. Nor is it an imposition hard to bear if one is asked to keep his muscles flexible or his eyes bright or his blood system pure by taking to yogic practices. At least blind self-interest should lead a man to this sort of physical culture. The tragedy of all of us is that having attained a miraculous, self-sustaining system of body, we choose to take it for granted and think that as long as it works smoothly, it is no part of our responsibility to maintain its machinery.

Depth psychology has shown that there is a form of psychic determinism which controls all our thoughts, actions and words. In fact, the revolution in modern psychological thought has infallibly led us to the conclusion that our conscious self is but a pygmy before the giant of our unconscious. The same truth was announced by the saints and seers of India as an intuitive truth, if not as a scientific maxim. The errors in man's personality go on multiplying in the process of living. Rectification of these errors can only be brought about if one addresses oneself to the task of understanding one's own mental structure.

It is here that the yogic system as enunciated by Patanjali, despite the shifting interpretations it has been subjected to, comes as a helping guide. The Patanjali system is in absolute concord with the principles of depth psychology. Freud said that the unconscious is mud; but it is also to be realized that out of that mud blossoms a lotus flower. The elaborate structure of human mind is definitely complicated but by relentless honesty with oneself, where no quarter is given and none taken, one can see oneself as clearly, or more so, as one sees oneself in a mirror. The yogic disciplines for the mind essentially direct one towards this sort of realization. It creates, in Milton's words, "a calm of mind, all passions spent". It is with this instrumentality, with minds and bodies as means to an end, that we can commence our spiritual journey to the Godhead.

Yogic philosophy offers no shortcuts to the Ultimate, it prescribes a long and a tortuous way. The very brevity of our lives makes it imperative for us to understand the urgency of our mission. There is no realization distinct from the understanding of ourselves and there is no ignorance different from neglect of our beings. Spiritual liberation dawns only when inner equipoise is attained by the rigours of the body and mind. And there cannot be any collective realization of divinity. Here each individual is left to himself. He is his own taskmaster and his own leader. He stands and falls by what he has decided to be. In the yogic path everything is incorruptible. Weakness of will, infirmity of decision, vacillations of mind may be equated with sin in puritan philosophy. They do not exist once the yogic discipline is imbibed in the self. The weak man is the strong man in embryo. The unspiritual is the spiritual storehouse in ignorance. Yoga philosophy delivers man from nescience to omniscience, from impotence to omnipotence, from finite to the infinite.

The plethora of spiritual movements has made spiritual choice difficult. Yoga is a heritage which comes to our rescue at a time when ambiguity surrounds philosophical thought. It is a heritage that needs to be preserved carefully and studied conscientiously in all its phases.

Yoga in Everyday Life

Yogasanas

THE YOGIC POSTURES

Yoga, as a science of living, is accepted in theory by quite a large number of thinking individuals. If we look closely at the development of the yogic movement in various parts of the world we will find that its application is largely confined to the physical aspects, viz. training in various asanas and pranayamas. This is indeed desirable as the physical well-being of an individual is essential for further spiritual development.

The first condition of human happiness is the possession of a sound body. A healthy body is an asset to enable man to work his way in everyday life. It is common knowledge that a sound mind, or a healthy mental condition, prevails in a healthy body. The yogasanas thus form the backbone of applied yoga.

The principal asanas are said to be eighty-four in number. A preliminary study, even theoretical, of the different postures will reveal that they are intended to serve the various parts of the body. Current systems of physical exercise help to build muscles and make an individual muscular. However, it is everyday experience that even a muscular man is unable to stand the strain and stress of life for a long time. It follows, therefore, that there is a constant and inescapable action of the mind on the body which the physical exercises are unable to tackle. Herein lies the main difference between asanas and physical exercise. The asanas are not only aids to keeping the physical system healthy and strong but they also help in an imperceptible way, with the assistance of their counterpart, pranayama, to build up a mental resistance to disease. They take into account various parts of the body and joints, and form in themselves a complete nerve toning system. The entire physical organism is dependent upon the nervous system, and unless the nerves are kept fit and nourished, the mere building up of muscles will not be of any use. Furthermore, the regular practice of asanas in daily life does not entail great strain upon the physical energy and time of an individual. A person with a weak constitution can also be admitted into an asana course, under proper guidance.

It may be of interest to note that many asanas are named after birds or animals, for example, *mayurasana* (the peacock pose), *shashankasana* (hare pose), *bhujangasana* (cobra pose) etc. If we try to understand the implications of the asanas they might give an interesting clue. After a day's work the body is fatigued, and our common belief is that it will be rested by assuming the horizontal position in which we sleep. How do birds and animals rest? Nature has deprived them of the comfort of a horizontal position and yet they do rest. Therefore, the poses in which they stand or rest give the clue to the asanas. As mentioned before, asanas are not strenuous exercises but are recreational poses which refresh a tired body and give it the necessary energy to carry on the day's labour with comfort and ease.

It may be necessary to explain here that asanas do not entail exertion as other physical exercises do, nor do they require rich food to make the body healthy. As a matter of fact, the entire concept behind asanas is to keep the human body fit and active as long as it lasts.

Out of the eighty-four asanas, only about twenty are important. They have been divided into the following five categories.

Postures for meditation

Padmasana (lotus pose)
Siddhasana (adept's pose)
Sukhasana (pleasant pose)
Swastikasana (auspicious pose)

Inverted postures

Sarvangasana (shoulderstand pose)
Halasana (plough pose)
Sirshasana (headstand pose)

Supine posture

Shavasana (corpse pose)

Face-down postures

Bhujangasana (serpent pose)
Shalbhasana (locust pose)
Dhanurasana (bow pose)
Mayurasana (peacock pose)

Miscellaneous postures

Paschimottanasana (forward bending stretch pose)
Vajrasana (thunderbolt pose)
Suptavajrasana (sleeping thunderbolt pose)
Shashankasana (hare pose)
Yogamudra (psychic union pose)
Baddhapadmasana (tied lotus pose)
Ardha matsyendrasana (half pose of Matsyendra)
Matsyasana (fish pose)

The technique of these asanas is described under each category indicating the benefits of individual asanas.

MEDITATION POSTURES

Padmasana

Spread a blanket and sit on it with legs stretched in front of you.

Then fold the right leg and place the foot on the left thigh. Similarly, fold the left leg and place the foot carefully on the right thigh.

Adjust the heels in such a way that they almost meet in front of the pubic bone and each foot presses the portion of the abdomen adjacent to it.

The position of the hands varies.

Some find it convenient to keep them on their respective knees while others place the right palm over the left palm, keeping both upturned and cupped.

While performing this asana, the head and spine must be held erect.

Benefits: Padmasana is an ideal asana for meditation. One can sit in this asana for hours together. The erect position of the spine helps the nerve flow along the spine and between the vertebrae to be carried out uninterruptedly. The erect spine also prevents the compression of the abdominal viscera and so frees the mind from the burden of the body. Padmasana tones up the coccygeal and sacral nerves. When a person sits in this posture for a long time, the lower portion of the body is compressed, interfering with the free circulation of blood. The coccygeal and sacral nerves get an extra supply of blood from the abdominal artery.

Siddhasana

Place one heel at the perineum and then place the other one above the genital organ.

Tuck the toes in between the calf and thigh.

Control the sense organs.

Keep the eyes fixed on one place and look at the space between the two brows.

Benefits: Siddhasana is said to give liberation and good results. The sense organs are to be controlled through control of mind. This asana is very important as this withdraws you from the world. The mind is controlled and merged in the Absolute if this asana is practised for long hours, persistently, for many years.

The therapeutic value of siddhasana is also considerable. It cures all diseases of the body by generating prana or life-force. Life-force runs throughout the organs of the body in the required proportions when the body and mind are set at rest.

Sukhasana

This is intended for those who are too stiff to perform the other meditation asanas.

In this case, after crossing the legs, raise the knees eight or nine inches above the ground.

Then pass a scarf or folded cloth round the small of the back and around the legs below the knees.

Knot it in front so that the weight of the knees is supported by the cloth.

The hands may then be put together palm to palm and rested on the cloth between the knees.

Swastikasana

Swastikasana means 'the cross pose'. The *swastika* is the sacred sign of the cross of Hindus. The cross is the most pious and sacred symbol of almost all the great religions of the world. Swastikasana is one of those four important asanas which are meant for meditational purposes.

Place the left foot between the calf and thigh of the right leg with the heel placed at the groin.

The right foot should be placed between the left calf and left thigh. Do not lean on one side.

It should be noted that swastikasana and siddhasana are similar except for the slight change in the position of the feet. Please note the change and practise it.

INVERTED POSTURES

Sarvangasana

Lie flat on the back.

Using the arms as levers, raise both legs to a vertical position.

Supporting the back with both hands, lift the trunk, hips and legs vertically, resting the elbows on the ground.

The chin may be pressed against the chest.

The shoulder portion of the back and neck touch the ground. Do not move the body, keep the legs straight.

Retain this pose as long as convenient.

When this asana is finished, bring down the legs very slowly without jerking.

Benefits: This asana nourishes the thyroid gland and promotes health in many ways. It supplies a large quantity of blood to the spinal column and keeps the spine elastic, which means everlasting youth. It helps in maintaining celibacy, checks wet dreams and is a powerful blood tonic and blood purifier. It tones the nerves and removes constipation as well as other gastro-intestinal disorders. This asana is also very useful for ladies as it relieves sterility and genito-urinary disorders.

Halasana

As in sarvangasana, lie flat on your back.

Keep the hands at the sides, placing them with the palms on the ground.

Raise the legs slowly without the help of the hands, do not bend the legs and the trunk.

Then slowly lower the legs over the head until the toes touch the ground.

The knees should be straight and close together.

The legs and thighs must be in one straight line, with the chin pressing the chest.

Breathe slowly through the nose.

You can also catch hold of the toes with the two hands.

In performing this asana there should be no jerking or strain.

When the asana is over, raise the legs slowly and bring them to the original position lying flat on the ground.

Benefits: The asana tones up the spinal nerves and the back muscles, preventing early ossification of the vertebral bones. Various sorts of muscular rheumatism, lumbago and sprain are cured. Obesity and chronic constipation, diabetes, and congestion and enlargement of the liver and spleen may also be cured by this asana.

Sirshasana

This is the king of all the asanas.

To perform it efficiently, spread a four-fold blanket and sit on the knees.

Interlock the fingers and make a triangular support on the ground. Place the crown of the head on the ground, so it is tightly wedged into this groove.

Slowly raise the legs till they are vertical.

Stand on the head for five seconds in the beginning and gradually increase the period.

Slowly bring the legs down.

This asana should be done slowly and carefully.

Avoid jerks while standing on the head.

Breathe slowly through the nose.

Benefits: By doing this asana you can sublimate sexual energy and maintain celibacy. The seminal energy is transmuted into spiritual energy and forms a spiritual force used for meditation. Memory increases. You will find real pleasure and exhilaration of spirit. The advantages derived are incalculable. It brightens the intellectual and psychic faculties. All diseases of the eyes, nose, throat, stomach, liver, spleen, lungs and kidneys are alleviated. Colic, deafness, gonorrhoea, diabetes, piles, asthma, consumption, syphilis etc., are eliminated. It augments the digestive fire. Utero-ovarian diseases, including sterility, are greatly helped.

SUPINE POSTURE

Shavasana

This is an asana for relaxation of all the nerves and muscles. It should be performed after all other asanas, as a last item.

Lie flat on the back keeping the hands on the ground by the sides, and stretch the legs quite straight.

Keep the heels and toes separated.

Close the eyes and breathe slowly.

Now relax all muscles, nerves and organs.

The relaxation process should start from the toes and proceed upwards, through all the organs, heart, chest and brain.

Benefits: Shavasana gives a rest to body, mind and soul. Relaxation is a very important factor in the regime of yoga exercises. The organs that are put under severe strain while performing asanas demand relaxation and rest. In shavasana, prompt and efficient relaxation is ensured.

FACE-DOWN POSTURES

Bhujangasana

Lie down flat on the ground, face downwards, and relax.

Place the palms flat on the floor under the shoulders.

Rest the forehead on the floor and relax the body.

Slowly raise the head and shoulders off the ground, bending the head as far back as it will go.

Try to raise the shoulders without using the arms, only utilizing the back muscles.

Now bring the arms into action and slowly bend the back as much as possible without strain until the arms are straight. Keep the navel as close to the ground as possible.

Hold as long as is comfortable.

Inhale while raising the body from the ground.

Breathe normally in the final pose.

Benefits: This asana is particularly for ladies to tone up the ovaries and uterus. It relieves ovarian disease. Child birth becomes normal and easy.

Shalabhasana

Lie on the ground, face downward, with the hands under the thighs.
Stretch the legs and straighten the arms.
Lift the legs, thighs and the lower portion of the abdomen.
While raising the legs, you must inhale, and retain the breath until you finish the asana.
Then exhale as you lower the legs.
This may be repeated 5 or 6 times.
Benefits: This asana bends the spine backward and it is a counterpose of sarvangasana and halasana. It gives a good exercise to the abdomen and relieves constipation. It tones up the abdominal organs, viz. liver, kidneys, etc., and removes several diseases of the stomach and bowels. The digestive fire is increased and dyspepsia removed.

Dhanurasana

This is a combination of bhujangasana and shalabhasana with the addition of catching the ankles with the hands. These three form one set of asanas. It is called dhanurasana, as the pose resembles a bow.
As in bhujangasana and shalabhasana, lie flat on the ground, face downwards, and relax all muscles.
Catch hold of the ankles with the hands and raise your chest and head, expanding the chest and keeping the arms and forelegs straight and stiff.
Retain this pose as long as is comfortable.
The whole body rests on the abdomen and gives it a good massage.
Benefits: This asana is useful in chronic constipation, dyspepsia and sluggish liver. It removes rheumatism of the legs, knee joints and hands. It reduces fat, energizes the digestive system and increases the appetite. It is a

blessing for people suffering from gastro-intestinal diseases. One who does halasana, mayurasana and dhanurasana will be full of energy, vigour and vitality.

Mayurasana

Kneel on the floor. Place the feet together and separate the knees.
Lean forward and place both palms between the knees on the floor, with the fingers pointing towards the feet.
Bring the elbows and forearms together.
Lean further forward and rest the abdomen on the elbows and the chest on the upper arms.
Stretch the legs backward so they are straight and together.
Tense the muscles and slowly elevate the trunk and the legs so that they are horizontal to the ground.
The whole body should then be balanced only on the palms of the hands.
Maintain the final pose for a short time without strain, then carefully return to the base position.
Exhale while raising the body, retain breath outside in final pose, inhale while lowering the body.
Benefits: This asana gives full exercise within a short time, and is wonderful for improving the digestion. It cures dyspepsia and diseases of the stomach and reduces enlargement of the spleen and liver. The lungs are properly toned. It improves the appetite, removes diseases caused by an excess of wind, cures diabetes and piles, and strengthens the muscles of the arms.

MISCELLANEOUS POSTURES

Paschimottanasana

Sit on the ground with the legs stretched out.
Bend the trunk forward and catch the toes with the index fingers.
There should be no jerking while bending.
Do not use any force.

After practice it should be possible to touch the knees with the forehead.

Retain the breath until you take the forehead back to its original position.

Breathe in when you have come back to the original position.

Those who cannot do the full posture may practise a preparatory posture with one leg and one hand, then with the other leg and hand alternately. This will be found easier.

After some practice, when the spine becomes elastic, the full pose can be done.

Benefits: This asana is excellent because it stimulates the gastric fire. It reduces fat on the abdomen and is specific for corpulence and enlargement of the spleen and liver. It stimulates the kidneys, liver, pancreas and increases the peristalsis of the intestines. It relieves constipation and removes sluggishness of the liver as well as dyspepsia and gastritis. Lumbago and all sorts of myalgia and other diseases of the back muscles are cured. This asana also cures piles and diabetes.

Vajrasana

The soles of the feet may be placed on both sides of the buttocks, calves touching the thighs.

The whole burden of the body is put on the knees and ankles. The knees should be kept quite close and the hands should rest straight on the knees.

Keep the trunk, neck and head in one straight line.

Benefits: Sitting in this asana, even after eating, is helpful for digestion. The stomach works vigorously. Myalgia in the knees, legs, toes and thighs disappears and sciatica vanishes. This asana alone can be done after eating.

Supta vajrasana

Sit in vajrasana. Bend backward, supported on the forearms and elbows.

The head touches the ground with the back arched. Place the hands on the thighs and make sure the knees stay fully on the ground.
Close the eyes and relax the body. Breathing should be slow and deep.
Benefits: Supta vajrasana has all the advantages of vajrasana with more pressure on the knees.

Shashankasana

Sit in the posture of vajrasana and raise both arms above your head in a straight line.
Breathe in and bend forward, releasing the breath slowly. The forehead and hands should reach the ground simultaneously.
Breathe in, come back slowly to the original posture.
Benefits: This posture cures dysentery, liver and kidney disorders. Backache is relieved.

Yogamudra

Sit in padmasana and place the palms on the heels.
Slowly bend forward while exhaling and touch the ground with your forehead or your chin.
Remain in this pose as long as you comfortably can while breathing in and out as usual.
Breathe out and come back to the former position as you breathe in.
You can also keep the hands at the back, catching hold of the left wrist with your right hand.
Benefits: This pose removes abdominal disorders and helps in concentration.

Baddhapadmasana

Sit in padmasana. Place the right hand behind the back and grasp the right big toe, with the left hand holding the left big toe.
It is easier to hold the big toes by breathing out and leaning slightly forward.

Benefits: Baddhapadmasana eliminates all diseases. If this asana alone is practised for half an hour, twice daily, no other asana need be done.

Ardha matsyendrasana

All the asanas described above are counterposes, bending the spine forward and backward which, alone, is not sufficient. The spine must be twisted and bent from side to side also. Only then can perfect elasticity be ensured. Ardha matsyendrasana serves this purpose well.

To perform this asana, sit with the legs straight in front of the body.

Place the right foot flat on the floor outside the left knee. Bend the left leg to the right and place the left heel against the right buttock.

Place the left arm outside the right leg, and with the left hand hold the right foot or ankle. The right knee should be as near as possible to the left armpit.

Turn the body to the right, placing the right arm behind the back. Twist the back and then the neck as far as possible without strain.

Remain in the final pose for a short time and then slowly return to the starting position.

Change the legs and repeat to the other side.

Matsyasana

Sit in padmasana.

Bend backward, supporting the body with the forearms and elbows, until the crown of the head touches the ground. Hold the big toes and rest the elbows on the floor. Arch the back as much as possible. Breathe deeply and slowly in the final pose.

This is one variation.

The other is that, after lying flat on the back, the head may rest on the crossed forearms.

When you have done this asana, slowly release the head with the help of the hands and sit up.

Benefits: This supplements sarvangasana. It destroys many diseases and removes constipation. It is also useful in asthma, consumption and chronic bronchitis.

Conclusion

1. Asanas should be practised in seclusion in a well ventilated room.
2. Asanas form an important part of the dynamic system of applied yoga. They can be practised by young and old with equal advantage.
3. Their demand on time is negligible, their benefits innumerable.
4. They effectively cure obesity by reducing fat. They ensure perfect digestion and cure constipation which happens to be a typical malady of the modern world.
5. They effectively lower high blood pressure.
6. They have great psychosomatic and psychophysiological potential.

Pranayama

THE BREATHING PROCESSES IN YOGA

Prana means the vitality of life which expresses itself through the various centres of the body. Its simple meaning is energy. Pranayama means the regulation or the control of prana (vital energy) in three stages: inhalation, retention and exhalation of breath.

Asana and pranayama are necessary for keeping the body healthy and fit. All of us without exception aspire for a healthy body. Nothing can be done in this world without a healthy body, neither day-to-day worldly duties, nor attainment of self-realization. An ailing person cannot even say his prayers properly. Everybody likes to have sound health, but for want of proper knowledge one has to suffer. The science of yoga teaches us how to improve and maintain good health.

Breath is life. One can live for some time without food but one cannot live without breathing. When we breathe in, air enters into our body. Air contains oxygen which is necessary for the body because of its life-giving property. The oxygen contained in air is the basis of all life. If there was no oxygen in the air, all living beings would be deprived of life. Oxygen is an element which helps burning. The process of gradual self-burning is what we call life. All the tissues of our body are constantly in a state of gradual combination with oxygen. This results in a continuous process of burning and destruction of a large number of tissues which produces heat in our body. In this way the temperature is maintained as is required for our existence.

Blood circulates continuously through our body through the circulatory system. There is a network of blood-circulating channels through our whole body. These are thin blood capillaries, thinner even than a hair. The walls of these capillaries are extremely thin and porous. The blood passes through these walls and reaches the tissues. The tissues take life-giving matter from it and throw out their own refuse into the blood channels. In this way oxygen passes on to the tissues and carbon dioxide produced by oxidation takes its place and is left in the blood. Thus blood returns to the heart carrying all the impurities of the system. The heart again pumps it out through small channels to the lungs where fresh air comes in contact with the lung tissues. Carbon dioxide is exhaled and oxygen is absorbed from the fresh air.

Every change in our body is a result of continuous chemical changes taking place in an infinite number of cells in the body. Whenever a muscle contracts or glands secrete, or even when we think of something, there is a chemical change in the corresponding organs of the body. By chemical changes we mean the process of oxidation. Oxygen that pervades the body, along with blood, combines with the compounds coming into contact with it and splits them up. This process also leads to the production of waste matters that are completely useless for our system and it becomes necessary to throw them out. These pass on as impure blood to the lungs, through the heart. From there they come out of our body with our breath through the air passages. This is the process of oxidation in a nutshell.

Good health is entirely dependent on the working of the internal mechanism, the glands and other organs of our system. One of the most important functions of our body is the process of inhalation (breathing in) and exhalation (breathing out). If this process is stopped, death is inevitable within a few minutes.

Therefore, it is essential that organs carrying out this important assignment should be perfectly healthy and strong. Very often, due to general debility of the respiratory organs, there is not satisfactory respiration and one becomes prey to several diseases of these organs: pneumonia, pleurisy, tuberculosis, colds, diseases of the throat, influenza and nasal troubles.

Pranayama is indispensable for getting rid of body toxins to avoid ailments and to strengthen the corresponding organs. One who practises pranayama becomes immune to such diseases.

Now let us try to explain what pranayama is. Prana means energy. The process of breathing in, breathing out, and holding the breath – a sum total of these three processes, that is to say, the three processes when combined – constitute full pranayama. People are generally afraid of pranayama. Several wrong notions prevail about it. For instance, it is said that those who practise pranayama have to pull air in and force it into places which may burst any moment and bring about death. This is far from the truth. We are not advocating anything here that may bring danger to life. That is not the purpose of yoga and has no place in this task. The reader should, therefore, cast off all such misgivings. There are, of course, certain advanced practices which the adepts teach only to properly qualified and deserving disciples and have them carried out in their own presence. But the course of pranayama explained here is simple, involves no danger, and can be practised by all.

Even normal respiration has three stages which go on all the time, whether we practise pranayama or not. These are: breathing in, breathing out and holding the breath for a while with ease. All types of pranayama consist of a particular combination of these three processes.

Benefits

Through practising pranayama the lungs become stronger and flexible. In the body, heat is generated which produces beneficial effects on general health. Oxygen is supplied to our body in large quantity. The greater the intake of oxygen, the greater is the quantity of carbon dioxide expelled.

Chemical changes brought about by physical exertion result in the break-up of matter within the body and consequent loss of energy. This loss is compensated by an increased supply of oxygen through pranayama. Pranayama also produces a healthy and invigorating effect on the brain and the nerves. It tones up the functioning of the brain, dormant centres in the smaller and greater brain are energized and latent potentialities are awakened. All round development of the pituitary and pineal glands is brought about by practising pranayama regularly.

Pranayama not only produces beneficial effects on the breathing system but also removes diseases of the ears, tongue, eyes and throat. Hoarseness, tonsillitis, eruption on the cheeks, deafness, etc., are all curable by pranayama. Like asana, pranayama has both preventative and curative effects. At first it gradually provides energy and strengthens different organs of the body. It bestows the power of resistance to disease. If at all some disease creeps in, it can be removed by the different processes of pranayama. For curative action in disease, pranayama should be learnt from those who are adepts and have practised it successfully.

Pranayama has its effect not only on the breathing mechanism but also on other organs of the body. The liver, kidneys, etc.., are all toned up, and by their brisk and vigorous activities the circulation of blood is accelerated, leading to oxidation with greater speed. Pranayama helps in expelling impurities from the body. It increases appetite, tones up the intestines and improves peristalsis, removing constipation. Pranayama is not only beneficial to the respiratory system but is also necessary for maintenance of general health and building up the whole system.

While practising vigorous pranayama, the mind becomes inactive and tranquil for some time. This provides some rest and relaxation. By practising retention of breath the mind becomes relaxed. There is no other way of bringing about relaxation of mind because thoughts always continue to come into it. While practising pranayama the mind becomes stationary and thoughts are exhausted. This is why pranayama is considered to be one of the best practices for concentration.

Through pranayama we gain control over the nerves. As soon as this is brought about, nervous tensions are minimized. Extraordinary strength and energy are obtained. Pranayama is a sure way to tone up the nervous system. Pranayama is a practice for casting impurities out from the human system. This is the process of purification of pranic channels.

Prana (life force) has a very close relation to the mind. As prana of the subtle pranic body (*pranamaya kosha*) is intrinsically linked to the other koshas, *annamaya* (food body), *manomaya* (mental body), etc., prana is influenced by thoughts, feelings, emotions etc., and they are influenced by prana.

TECHNIQUES OF PRANAYAMA

We shall now discuss the different kinds of pranayama and ways of practising them, as well as the application in the treatment of diseases.

There are three essentials of pranayama: asana, mudra and process. A small folded blanket is required. We should choose a place where there is a pure and calm atmosphere. Pranayama should not be practised in a dirty, impure, offensively smelling or smoky place. An open and well ventilated room, even in winter, is most appropriate for practising pranayama. One should practise it sitting on a folded blanket on the floor. The best time for practising pranayama is in the early hours of the morning.

Those who practise asana should first practise them after attending to morning duties, washing and bathing. Pranayama should be practised after asana. An important thing to remember is that pranayama should always be practised with empty bowels or at least four hours after taking meals. Practice of pranayama should be reduced in frequency during the summer and increased vigorously, but gradually, during the winter.

How should one sit for pranayama? The best postures are padmasana (lotus posture) and siddhasana (adept's pose). Those who can sit in padmasana should sit in that posture with a peaceful mind. One thing to be taken care of is that the spinal cord should remain straight and vertical. The head and the neck should also remain erect. One can sit in whatever posture one likes; the point to remember is that it should be quite comfortable so that there may be no necessity to change position during the practice.

The eyes will remain closed while doing pranayama. The right hand is free to manipulate the nose. The left hand should remain comfortably on or near the knee, or kept in the lap with the palm up.

While practising pranayama one has to close the nostrils. This is done with the right hand and the nose is held in a particular manner. One may hold the nose in any way one likes but the correct procedure is as follows: when the left nostril is to be closed it should be done with the fourth (ring) finger of the right hand, and when the right one is to be closed it should be done with the right thumb.

Pranayama can be practised by everyone without exception. In fact, all living beings are breathing in and out, in other words, are practising pranayama. So, a few simple and easy types of pranayama can be safely practised even by ailing persons. Those who are too weak can do a light course lying in bed. Such persons should fill their lungs with air very slowly, the air should be evacuated similarly. We are all doing this consciously or unconsciously. Pranayama techniques only teach us how to do it correctly.

Let us now deal with various kinds of pranayama and how to practise them. There are three stages of pranayama viz. *pooraka*, *rechaka* and *kumbhaka*.

When we breathe in or inhale, this is called pooraka, and when we breathe out or exhale, it is known as rechaka. When we hold the breath, it is said to be kumbhaka.

Kumbhaka is of two kinds. To hold the breath after breathing in is antar kumbhaka, and to hold the breath outside after exhalation is termed bahir kumbhaka. These will be the terms used hereafter and should be borne carefully in mind – pooraka for breathing in, rechaka for breathing out, antar kumbhaka for holding the breath inside after pooraka, and bahir kumbhaka for holding the breath outside after rechaka.

Important pranayamas are: *sukhpoorvaka, samaveta, sahita, nadi shodhana, bhramari, ujjayi, sheetali, sheetkari, bhastrika, suryabheda, kewali, plawini and chaturtha.*

Simple or sukhpoorvaka

One thing to remember here is that pooraka is to be performed through the same nostril which performs rechaka. Rechaka and then pooraka can be done with one nostril but pooraka and rechaka should not be done with the same nostril at one time. If one nostril performs pooraka, the other nostril is to perform rechaka. This will mean automatically that pooraka will be performed by the same nostril which performs rechaka. Through practising this, the intensity of the flow of air through both nostrils is equalized. All the benefits of pranayama are derived from this practice. Those who have congested nostrils while sleeping are freed of this trouble. Those who are susceptible to coughs must practise this daily for at least five to seven minutes.

Practise pranayama with a cheerful mind and you will derive extraordinary benefits. Practising pranayama half-heartedly, carelessly or in a state of hurry can be detrimental.

Practice

Sit in padmasana or siddhasana. Make your mind calm. Sit calmly for a minute, compose yourself, and prepare yourself for pranayama.

Now lift your right hand and make it ready to hold the nostrils.

First close the right nostril and breathe in through the left only.

Take in as much breath as you can, very slowly, and when the lungs are filled with air, close the left nostril.

Open the right one and breathe out slowly.

As soon as the full breath is out, breathe in fully again with the same (i.e. right) nostril, close it, and open the left nostril and exhale slowly.

This makes one round.

The process is like this – pooraka with the left nostril and rechaka with the right, then pooraka with the right and rechaka with the left.

This completes one round.

Then again pooraka with the left and so on.

Repeat this 15–20 times.

Samaveta pranayama

This should be done after practising sukhpoorvaka (all the rules are the same for this pranayama).

Practice

Pooraka through both nostrils simultaneously.

Take as much air as possible into the lungs.

Hold the breath for a while, say for 1–3 seconds, and then do rechaka with both nostrils.

Then again pooraka with both nostrils slowly.

Then rechaka the same way.

Sahita pranayama

In this pranayama, kumbhaka has been added to the pooraka and rechaka processes.

Remember, there is no need for a forced performance. You have to hold the breath only as long as you can very comfortably do so without experiencing any difficulty. Everybody can hold the breath for some time. As you advance in your practice, flexibility of the lungs will increase along with the power to retain the breath.

Practice

Do pooraka as stated above in samaveta pranayama.
Close both nostrils and hold the breath (kumbhaka).
Hold it as long as you can with ease and comfort.
Then breathe out slowly with both nostrils.
This will complete 1 round.

Nadi shodhana pranayama

This pranayama is similar to sahita pranayama, the only difference being that you have to fix the duration of pooraka, kumbhaka and rechaka to the ratio 1:4:2, and breathe through alternate nostrils.

Nadi shodhana pranayama is of three categories: *uttama* (the best), *madhyama* (medium) and *kanishta* (inferior). All should be learnt slowly and cautiously.

- Pooraka 12, kumbhaka 48, rechaka 24 – yogis call this kanishta pranayama.
- Pooraka 16, kumbhaka 64, rechaka 32 – this is called madhyama pranayama.
- Pooraka 20, kumbhaka 80, rechaka 40 – this is called uttama pranayama.

This pranayama improves the pulse and casts off all impurities. By attaining perfection in this pranayama the body becomes light. One gains full control over the nerves and body.

Practice

Sit in any comfortable asana.
Breathe in through the left nostril while counting 1 to 4 mentally.
Retain the breath while counting 1 to 16 by closing both nostrils.
The retention should be so timed that it takes 4 times the time taken for inhalation.

Then exhale with the right nostril counting mentally from 1 to 8.

Repeat this practice by doing pooraka with the right nostril, then kumbhaka, and then rechaka with the left nostril, with the ratio thc same as before, i.e. 4:16:8.

Bhramari pranayama

This is a very easy pranayama. Anybody can practise it well from the very first day. Through practice of this pranayama, all diseases of the throat are radically alleviated. The larynx becomes strong, the voice sweet. Bhramari should be practised in a solitary place late at night or early in the morning.

Practice

Sit in any comfortable asana with a composed mind.

Close both ears with the first (index) finger.

Take a full breath slowly and hold just for a short while and breathe out with a humming sound like that of a bee. This humming sound should continue till the breathing out is completed.

The mouth should remain closed but the teeth should be slightly apart.

The tongue should not move, while the mind should remain fully concentrated on the humming sound. The continuity and uniformity of this humming sound should not break till the end.

Ujjayi pranayama

This pranayama is most beneficial to those who have enlarged tonsils, or those who are very sensitive to cold and suffer from cough, and those who often get attacks of influenza or bronchitis. It is also beneficial to students of vocal music. It is often seen that their voices becomes hoarse due to excessive practise of music. Sometimes this trouble comes suddenly. If they practise ujjayi pranayama regularly their throats will always remain healthy and their voice will become sweet and melodious.

If sufferers of tonsillitis are asked to practise this pranayama they will be cured. It also produces good effects on diseases of the ear, nose and throat and brings down high blood pressure.

Practice

Sit in any comfortable asana and close your eyes.

The mouth should remain closed and all breathing should take place through the nose.

While inhaling, a sound similar to that of a snoring baby should be produced in the throat.

To produce this sort of sound, the underside of the tongue is kept touching the palate (*khechari mudra*) and the breath is inhaled.

Pooraka is done with a sound similar to that of an idling steam engine, and after keeping the breath inside for a while, rechaka follows with the same sound.

A hissing sound should invariably be produced. This should be done 10–12 rounds daily.

Sheetali pranayama

This pranayama should be practised for curing diseases of the throat and tongue. This has good effects on a sore throat and tonsils. Sheetali, sheetkari and ujjayi should be practised for curing stammering. If there are eruptions on the face, or the tongue is dry and cracked, this pranayama should be practised regularly every day.

By attaining perfection in sheetali pranayama, one can control hunger and thirst. Cough, biliousness, constipation and indigestion are all cured. This pranayama is bliss for yogis.

Practice

Sit in any comfortable asana and put out the tongue and twist it so as to form a channel or a round tube.

Breathe in. The breath should be taken in slowly and gently so as to fill up the lungs completely.

Then do rechaka through the nose.

While doing rechaka, the tongue should be taken in.

Again pooraka with the tongue taken out in the shape of a tube and then rechaka is to be repeated through the nose, with the tongue inside.

Practise 8–10 rounds every day.

Sheetkari pranayama

In this pranayama, there is only pooraka through the mouth and rechaka through the nose. There is no kumbhaka. This pranayama produces soothing and beneficial effects in diseases of the mouth (including mouth ulcers), throat and nose.

Practice

The tongue should be inverted, its fore part touching the palate, and the upper teeth should be kept tight with the corresponding teeth of the lower jaw.

The lips remain open.

Breathe in through the mouth with a hissing sound.

The teeth and tongue will not move.

The open space by the sides of the tongue provide enough room for the air to pass through.

After pooraka, do rechaka through the nose.

Repeat this 8–10 rounds a day.

Bhastrika pranayama

Bhastrika pranayama is of paramount importance. However, those having a weak heart or lungs, or those who are ill should not practise this. People in normal health should practise this pranayama regularly.

It is important to note that in bhastrika pranayama the intensity of the pressure of air going in and coming out should remain equal. Another thing to be remembered is that there should not be unusual pressure on the walls of the nose. It should work like a bellows and should remain just normal.

Twenty times fast pooraka-rechaka, then kumbhaka and then in the end rechaka, constitutes one complete round of bhastrika pranayama. This can be practised up to 5 rounds at a time. Rest a while after each round. This pranayama can be practised both in the morning and evening.

Bhastrika pranayama cures asthma and other respiratory troubles, but for this purpose it should be practised under the guidance of an expert. Weak lungs are rejuvenated and strengthened.

During the practice of this pranayama, a greater supply of oxygen is made to enter the body and a greater amount of carbon dioxide is thrown out. Blood is purified and there is a greater and faster supply of blood throughout the body. Let us now learn how to practise it.

Practice

Breathe in slowly and do full pooraka through both nostrils, followed by rechaka, expanding and contracting the abdomen rhythmically.

The mouth should remain closed.

After doing this 4 or 5 times, the rapidity of pooraka and rechaka should be gradually increased so that, after 10 or 12 times, the breath should start flowing like a blacksmith's air bag. (Bhastrika means bellowing.)

After performing this pooraka-rechaka combined process about 20 times without a break, take a long pooraka and stop with antar kumbhaka.

Stay in this state of antar kumbhaka as long as you comfortably can.

After that, breathe out and empty the lungs slowly and gradually.

Rest for a while, taking normal breaths.

Then repeat this pranayama.

You can count numbers while in the state of kumbhaka.

Kewali pranayama

Concentration of mind is attained through the practice of this pranayama.

Practice

In kewali pranayama, breathing in and breathing out are carried on as follows.

Along with breathing in you have to pronounce the word *so* mentally, and similarly, while breathing out you have to pronounce the word *ham* mentally.

In this way, mental pronunciation of *soham* should be continued.

Plawini pranayama

This cures all bowel troubles. The power of digestion improves and it helps in effecting a cure for hysteria.

Practice

Sit in any comfortable asana and go on drinking in the air, as you drink water, until the stomach is filled with air. Then pass the air out through the mouth in such a way that all air taken in comes out immediately.

Chaturtha pranayama

The time taken in doing pooraka and rechaka and their frequency are maintained equally in this pranayama. In order to maintain equal frequency and duration of pooraka and rechaka, help is taken in the form of counting numbers of mantra japa.

Practice

Breathe in while counting numbers, say 1 to 4 or up to any number.

Breathe out counting up to the same number with the same speed.

After some time, pronounce the mantra mentally in place of numbers.

If you mentally pronounce *Om* 4 times while breathing in, you should likewise repeat *Om* 4 times while breathing out. Practise this for 10–15 minutes daily.

Conclusion

Different kinds of pranayama have been explained so far. It is not necessary to practise all of them daily. Their practice should be gradually increased day by day. Ten minutes regular practice is sufficient for maintaining good health. It is for one's own judgement to decide which pranayama one should practise, depending on one's capacity.

Sweat coming out of the body during pranayama should be rubbed into the body. Cast off any misapprehensions you have in your mind and practise three or four pranayamas regularly every day. You will realize and appreciate their beneficial effects for yourself.

Bandhas

FLEXIONS FOR CONTROL OF INVOLUNTARY ORGANS

Bandhas are internal flexions and are the yogic technique of controlling and exercising the involuntary organs which are connected with nerves in the body. Their effects on the nervous plexes (groups of nerves) are salutary. They possess a remarkable curative value in many physical ailments concerning organic and functional disorders. Their psychological and physiological utility is remarkable.

In yoga, four bandhas were known and practised down the ages. They are *jalandhara*, *uddiyana*, *moola* and *maha bandha*. The technique of practising the bandhas is described below.

Jalandhara bandha

Inhale, hold the breath and bend the head forward. Press the chin against the chest and contract the throat muscles. Raise the head before exhaling. It can also be done with the breath retained outside.

Benefits: Jalandhara bandha controls the function of the thyroid gland, on which development of the whole body depends. This bandha has considerable curative value in disorders of the throat.

Uddiyana bandha

Sit in a meditative pose with palms on the knees and knees resting on the floor. Close the eyes and relax the whole body. Exhale deeply and retain the breath outside. Perform jalandhara bandha. Then contract the abdominal muscles as far as possible inwards and upwards. This is the final position. Hold this lock for as long as the breath can be retained outside. Then slowly release the abdominal muscles, jalandhara and inhale.

This is known as uddiyana bandha. Literally, uddiyana means to fly. Allow the abdominal muscles to fly up into the cavity of the chest.

Benefits: Uddiyana cures constipation and stimulates digestive fire, removes intestinal disorders and worms, and activates the liver and the kidneys. It regulates the function of the adrenal glands and hypogastric plexus.

Moola bandha

Sit in siddhasana or siddha yoni asana.

Inhale, retain the breath and contract the muscles in the region of the perineum.

Hold comfortably for the length of the breath.

Exhale.

Benefits: Strengthens the sphincter muscle. Disorders of the urinary tract and associated sexual organs are relieved and nerves and muscles toned.

Maha bandha

Sit in siddhasana or siddha yoni asana.

Simultaneously perform jalandhara, uddiyana and moola bandhas, holding the breath outside.

Benefits: Controls the secretions of the endocrine glands. Bestows good health and vigour.

Mudras

TECHNIQUES TO REVITALIZE GLANDS AND ORGANS

Mudras are techniques for activating the glandular functioning and the dormant psychic power centres, and have two aspects of utility. One is the physical side and the other is the mental. They are the techniques for controlling the involuntary organs which are connected with the nerves of the body. Mudras help one approach nearer to the inner conscious energy. Yogis or aspirants in yoga can never progress unless they have mastered the mudras. It has been found from experience that the mudras are very effective and beneficial. Important mudras are described below.

Shambhavi mudra

Direct your eyes towards the middle of the eyebrows and meditate on your own self.

This is known as *shambhavi mudra*.

Benefits: This practice gives control over thoughts and the breath. The mind is suspended within for a short time and entrance into the psychic world becomes easier. It is a very important technique for passing into the astral domain. Insomnia is cured by the practice of this mudra.

Nabho mudra

Nabha means sky. *Nabho mudra* is to direct the tongue towards the palate while looking at the space between the eyebrows. Nabho mudra is perfect when you achieve shambhavi and twist the tongue backwards and touch the palate.

Benefits: Mudras are beneficial to physical health. They are also preparatory exercises useful for developing spiritual powers. Nabho mudra is very mysterious practice which cures several diseases. When the tongue is turned upward and that position is maintained for several minutes, the submaxillary glands begin to secrete. This secretion should be gulped down. This salivary juice is very good for the appetite and maintenance of youth. Touching the palate with the tongue is also very important as there is a special yogic centre in the palate region.

Kaki mudra

Shape your mouth like a crow's beak and inhale slowly and gradually.

Exhale through the nose.

Benefits: This mudra stimulates the digestive secretions and eliminates many diseases.

Khechari mudra

Close the mouth. Roll the tongue backwards so that the normally lower surface touches the upper palate. Try to bring the tongue tip as far back as possible without strain. Retain for as long as possible and perform ujjayi pranayama. If discomfort arises, relax the tongue for a few seconds.

Benefits: With practice, the tongue will automatically ascend into the sinuses to stimulate many vital nerve centres in the brain. This gives extensive health benefits to the body. This practice needs patience and perseverance. One who perfects khechari does not suffer from hunger, thirst, tiredness or langour. Used in kundalini awakening.

Bhujangini mudra

Drink in air through the mouth and draw it into the stomach.

Hold for a short time and then expel the air by belching.

Benefits: This helps eliminate disorders of the stomach.

Conclusion

All these mudras bestow power and health on the regular practitioner. All of them are very important and very effective. If you practise them you will know their merits yourself; there is no proof more convincing than one's own experience. The benefits of mudras are undoubted. They are scientific and aim at correcting the organic disorders of the body. Mudras encourage awareness of vital energy currents (prana), mental, psychic and spiritual attitudes.

Hatha Yoga

A PANACEA FOR BODILY ILLS

Hatha yoga does not denote yogasanas. *Ha* stands for *surya* (sun) or pingala nadi or vital energy (prana). *Tha* stands for *chandra* (moon) or ida nadi or mental energy. Hatha yoga is meant to effect harmony between the discordant principles in the sympathetic and parasympathetic nervous systems. Sushumna nadi is the central nervous system. If purity, peace, harmony and strength prevail in the nervous system, the psychic centres become awakened.

Hatha yoga consists of six purificatory processes: neti, dhauti, basti, kapalbhati, trataka and nauli. These are collectively known as the shatkarmas. These practices of hatha yoga help in the elimination of accumulated toxins from the body. All these practices should be learned under expert guidance.

Neti

The first of the practices in hatha yoga is neti. While doing neti, the nasal membrane is treated so that the sensation vibrates throughout the brain and awakens its entire system, thus removing all congestion and depression.

Ladies in India put a few drops of lukewarm oil into the nasal passages as a treatment for colds. The oil causes sneezing, removes congestion of the passages and lubricates the mucus membrane. In facial paralysis, sniffing ghee through the nose is found to be extremely helpful.

Practice

Neti with water (*jala neti*) is practised with a special neti lota. Fill the lota with tepid water and add half a teaspoon of salt.

Breathe through the open mouth.

Insert the the spout into the left nostril and tilt the head to the right so the water runs freely out of the right nostril. Repeat through the right nostril.

Dry the nose thoroughly by doing bhastrika pranayama, but do not use force.

Benefits: Milk can be used after jala neti, in the same way. It has been observed to relieve eye sores, cerebral depression and nasal infections. Colds, infections and inflammation of the mucus membrane will be removed.

Sutra neti

Doctors normally advise cauterization of the nasal passage, but neti is a simple method to cure nasal diseases.

Practice

Take a rubber catheter, pass it through the nostril, and take out one end from the mouth, holding the bigger end outside the mouth firmly.

You can also rub it by moving it to and fro for a while. Repeat for the other nostril. This is *sutra neti*.

Dhauti

Dhauti with water is one such method by which the stomach is given a thorough wash by means of warm saline water. The whole process consists of drinking about two litres of saline water and vomiting it all out by means of rubbing the root of the tongue with the fingers. However, care should be taken regarding the diet after this practice, because wrong food will undo the good effect. This practice is called *kunjal kriya* when done on an empty stomach.

Varisara dhauti or *shankhaprakshalana*, is a complete system of internal cleansing. It is done by drinking as much as five litres, or even more, of warm saline water. The entire process consists of drinking the water, performing special asanas and the evacuation of stool. This should be learned under expert guidance.

Vastra dhauti is a method of washing and exciting the stomach by swallowing a long bandage while holding onto one end, practising nauli, then pulling out the bandage. Though a panacea for asthmatics, it is not advisable to practise it daily.

Vatsara dhauti is a specialized technique of gulping air into the stomach during plawini pranayama, retaining it for some time in the stomach, and then evacuating the entire load of air either through the anus or through the mouth. This has the effect of throwing out impure gases from the system.

Nauli

Sustained practice of agnisar leads to uddiyana. When uddiyana is fairly perfected one can take to nauli very easily. It is not possible to learn nauli from this book. This practice tones all abdominal muscles.

Basti

Basti may be called the yogic enema. In this technique the practitioner sucks water in through the anus by doing nauli and again evacuates the same through the anus. The colon is cleaned and purified.

Kapalbhati

Just as an exhaust fan removes bad air from a room, the brain is also shaken by the process of kapalbhati.

Practice

Perform a number of rapid respirations, with the emphasis on exhalation.

The inhalation should be spontaneous without effort, only exhalation should be gently forced.

Exhale deeply, hold the breath outside and take your awareness to chidakasha.

Benefits: This removes certain cerebral tensions.

Trataka

There are various methods of trataka. One can hold trataka on water, fire, earth, sky, air, a dot, light, and the like. Each has its own cluster of significant attributes. Certain practices improve the eyesight while others are helpful in removing certain cerebral congestions and reviving memory.

Practice

Using a candle flame at eye level, sit an arm's length away from it.

Close the eyes and make the body completely steady.

Open the eyes and gaze (do not stare) at the tip of the wick of the candle flame. If the eyes feel strain then close them completely.

Rest them for one minute, gazing internally at the after image.

Do not blink the eyes.

Continue this practice for up to 10 to 15 minutes.

Mechanics of Meditation

Japa Yoga

HAMMERING THE UNCONSCIOUS

The word japa in Sanskrit means repetition of the name of God. In all the religions of the world the practice of the repetition of the name of the Divine has been prescribed as a daily ritual. Japa has been recognized to be the most powerful expedient enabling an aspirant to reach those regions of final beatitude and bliss for which all human beings aspire at one stage or other. Therefore, in this modern age where human beings have lost all their sense of values and are going the wrong way, one of the most potent and affecting redeemers from the sorrows of this world is japa, the repetition of God's name. Japa is thus regarded and recognized as one of the easiest methods for liberation from bondage.

Patanjali, the great exponent of yoga, in explaining the last element of devotion to God, declares that the sacred syllable *Om* is the symbol of the Almighty Being, and an aspirant seeking illumination should not only repeat this *mantra* but also contemplate on its meaning. It is clear, therefore, that japa has been prescribed and regarded as a sort of yoga practice and that is why the expression 'japa yoga' is used while discussing this technique. It also implies that there must be some scientific method whereby it may yield some definite result. Here we shall try to explain some of the main features of the technique of japa yoga and the prescribed method of practising it.

What is japa yoga?

Since japa implies repeating some sacred formula there must be such a definite formula, and that formula is called a mantra. Etymologically, mantra is something which, when repeated and contemplated upon, enables the practitioner to reach his goal. So a mere mechanical repetition of the mantra is ruled out. The practitioner has not only to comprehend its inner meaning fully but also to meditate upon it.

In yoga, therefore, great importance is assigned to the practice of japa. It is a method of spiritual communion through the repetition of the mantra. By continued repetition you create certain a vibration in your system. The recitation of the mantra purifies the physical organism and also fills the mind with spiritual vitality. Japa frees one from a host of mental vagaries and problems. According to realized saints, the mantra gives perfect knowledge of God and is the best medium for communion with God.

Preparatory stages

How should one begin practising japa? The normal requirements are that one should sit in a comfortable posture in a quite place with a serene mind. Laziness or lethargy, yawning, mental agitation, drowsiness or any sensation of hunger or thirst should be avoided. There should be no bodily movement, eyes should be closed and no part of the body below the waist should be touched. Since mantra japa is treated as a yoga practice, mere repetition of the mantra without inner sanctity, or with diffused consciousness, will not be of any avail. The technique of japa is calculated to release the latent power within us, and it is because of this that, in yoga, japa is treated as a part of *kriya yoga*. It is said that mere mental or verbal repetition of the name without following the prescribed method bears no fruit. The whole effect drains away like water from a broken vessel. In other words, before a spiritual aspirant sits for japa he should necessarily create within himself an atmosphere of purity.

Japa should then follow. The mantra has to be repeated neither too slowly nor too fast, for here again the practitioner is cautioned that too lethargic a repetition of the mantra will lead to physical ailments and too rapid a repetition to a loss of all benefit.

We request you to proceed with a conviction that in japa yoga the mantra which is recited is very powerful, and that it confers powers. This fact has been amply demonstrated. It is within common experience that various maladies are removed by japa. Curing snake-bite by mantra is not an unusual sight in India. Also, hypertension, fever, hysteria and blood pressure are cured by japa. It evidently goes to show that there is a divine power latent in mantra japa which is released through faith and willpower.

Our hypothesis is that the real power is in the mantra itself. Just as the explosive power latent in a cartridge remains unreleased unless hammered by a rifle pin, likewise the divine power in any mantra also remains unreleased unless approached through the practice of japa with full faith and willpower. It is also necessary to aim the mantra with one-pointedness. When the mantra is awakened and becomes potent, its presiding deity or the invisible power comes into operation.

According to the science of occultism, in every mantra there are invisible powers and deities hidden beyond our normal perception. If anyone argues that a mantra is simply an arrangement of syllables, nobody should believe him, because his view is scientifically untenable. Theosophists like Leadbeater, Annie Besant and Madame Blavatsky have clearly stated in their writings that a mantra is totally different from a mere alphabetical congregation. If you come across the book *Garland of Letters* by Sir John Woodroffe, you will realize that a mantra or any occult syllable has a secret power and meaning. All mantras, whether intelligible or not, were uttered by saints after full realization. Thus the supermental expressions came to be known as mantras. Mantras composed by grammarians are not mantras, but a grouping of letters. Unless one sees a mantra in realization, he cannot formulate it. So mantra is a revealed product, not simply an arrangement of syllables.

You must have read in the Bible about 'the word of God'. Everyone trying to reach the roof of the head is given a 'word', which is called the mantra. Since receiving the divine sound or mantra, these saints have, in succession, given them to their disciples. If you want evidence or testimony, you will find it in all holy scriptures of the world that the word was always revealed.

All mantras belong to two categories commonly known as *sakam* and *nishkam*. When repeated without self-interest, it is nishkam japa. This forms a part of pure devotion, while sakam japa is repetition of a mantra to achieve a particular end, for instance, to cure oneself of an obstinate illness.

Those who do japa of sakam mantra for curing a sick person should do the mantra practice according to the rules laid down in the scriptures. There are many rules and regulations regarding the type of *mala* or rosary, the system of doing japa, purificatory rites, etc.

If you want to do nishkam japa, for spiritual upliftment alone, there is no rule as such. You can practise japa either before or after a bath and at any place and time. There is no regulation of direction, time, place and process.

Then again, every mantra has twofold usefulness. When it becomes the *ishta* (desired) mantra, one has to do a certain number of beads daily. When we repeat our ishta mantra, either daily or occasionally, it forms a part of our prayer.

There are four stages in the process of practising japa. The first is verbal, that is loud chanting of the mantra. The second is repetition in whispers. This is more powerful than the first one. The second system is not for beginners. If they take to it, they will find the mind running here and there. The third is the mental *manasik* japa in which you have to meditate on the mental vibrations of the mantra. You have to feel the mantra mentally, no audible or whispering sound is to be made. This third system of repetition of japa is definitely more powerful than the first and the second. This method too is not for beginners. It is for those who have advanced in the practice of japa. The fourth is *ajapa*, which has been separately dealt with in detail later in the book. Though each is superior to the other, aspirants should practise japa in all its four stages.

Japa should either be done in padmasana (lotus posture) or in siddhasana (adept's posture) or sukhasana (pleasant posture). One should be able to sit comfortably in any of these postures for at least ten minutes to practise japa.

Before sitting for japa it is beneficial to say a few prayers. If you do not do so, with progressive introversion, the tensions due to physical or mental strain will materialize during the process of japa in the form of visions. To avoid drowsiness and dreams do *baikhari* (audible) japa.

When you roll the beads, you should be alert and mindful. Concentration is not suspension of mind, nor even one-pointedness of mind or total attention. But it implies awareness. During japa, hypnotized consciousness and mechanical repetition are checked. The mind is very cunning. It knows many tricks. If you go to an expert for analysis, you will find your conscious mind thinking of hell, whereas the subconscious mind is thinking of heaven; the conscious mind thinking of purity, and the subconscious mind thinking of impurity. In order to have a grip over all the dimensions of consciousness, using the beads will be very helpful if its traditional methods are not ignored.

The use of a mala

The mala has an important place in this practice. A mala with 108 beads and a principal bead is usually used for japa. The mala actually serves as an aid or instrument for this yogic practice. Normally a *sadhaka* provides himself with a rosary but, where one has no mala available, counting the japa on the fingertips can also be resorted to. The mala, or counting the japa on the fingertips, has been prescribed because considerable importance has been attached to counting during japa. The mala should be made of *tulsi*, *rudraksha* seeds or crystal.

A mala is necessary for japa. All great saints have prescribed the mala for japa. The Christians have the rosary. It is always good and helpful to have a mala. We must not hold conservative views or submit ourselves to scepticism in such vital matters.

There is a definite way of holding the mala while doing japa. We use only three fingers: the thumb, the third and the fourth fingers, and totally avoid the second and fifth fingers. This is the first rule. The second rule is that we do not rotate it forwards, we rotate it backwards. According to the third rule of japa, we must not cross the *sumeru* (principal bead). This is a very good rule, since it avoids chances of absent-mindedness, mechanical rotation and the like. The most important point is constant observation and bead-to-bead awareness of mantra and the second-to-second process of japa.

You can meditate on the form of the mantra, sound vibrations of the mantra, or guardian deity of the mantra, or else you can be aware that you are meditating. You must be aware of the mantra or the process of japa, and also the form of the ishta devata either with open or closed eyes. You can do trataka at the time of japa without blinking your eyelids.

In conclusion, let us summarize japa yoga. Japa is repetition of any mantra on a mala. The principal bead is called sumeru. You can call it the point of revival in terms of psychology. While doing japa on the mala, you should not touch the mala with your second and fifth fingers. Hold the mala closely and at the level of your biological heart or on your knee. When you complete the mala and arrive at the principal bead, you should be careful not to cross it but reverse the mala and go back the same way.

So remember these three points in japa:

1. Each mantra has a deity. Do not doubt or reason. You have no authority to deny this unless you can logically prove that it is not so.

2. Mantra can be awakened.
3. Through the awakened mantra we can fulfil our divine aspirations.

After the mantra provides you with peace and prosperity, can you forget God? No. Devotion grows slowly. Do japa and maintain awareness.

Trataka

CRYSTAL GAZING

During the process of meditation, when the meditating self and object of meditation combine and merge into one, it is called meditation. Perfect concentration is attained only when the three merge into each other. Perfection of concentration is meditation.

The form of truth is released in the stage of perfect concentration. All knowledge resides within the individual, but it does not come up to the brain because external objects exercise so great an influence over us, that they cover the things within us and we are not able to perceive them. The mind of man, through all the hours of day and night, revolves round the objects of the world with or without reason. Day in and day out man schemes to secure these material things. Thus, so long as the mind is extrovert it cannot be introvert. Since childhood our mind is used to being extrovert. It thus acquires bad habits and is not willing to think of anything other than worldly things.

With such an extrovert mind it is not possible to acquire knowledge. That is why certain practices are indicated. External objects are also used as an aid to awaken this power. For the power of concentration one has to take a material object also. Moreover, soul force is revealed through language, music, and other activities.

Trataka is one such practice, the efficacy of which has been long established. Through this practice one can even predict past and future events. This, of course, is a difficult sadhana for attaining perfection. Some progress can, however, be made by one who will practise sincerely.

Crystal gazing

Crystal stone is found in old rocks. It is the essence of the rocks. Just as coal is found in a coal mine, so also crystal is found in mountains and rocks. It is a transparent stone, more transparent and clear than water. Objects are seen as clearly through it as reflected on a mirror. It is also called *sphatik mani*. In very old mountains they form in a round circular shape. This stone is not easily available today. But if a seeker happens to get it, it should be used for sadhana.

The crystal stone should be kept in a separate room. It should be kept at eye level at a distance of one foot. Bathe the crystal with pure water and clean it with a clean piece of cloth. Thereafter, one should gaze at it steadily without a flicker of the eyelids. The eyes should be steady. To begin with, this should be done for five minutes first and extended to half an hour later. Continue gazing at some point in the crystal (steadily) in such a way that one does not see anything except the crystal. This practice should be continued for a month or more.

The second stage will then follow more easily. In this stage you should gaze at the crystal but without the consciousness that you are doing so. It is a stage similar to that in which, at the time of sleep, the consciousness of seeing does not remain. But there is a lot of difference between the stage of sleep and this practice. In this practice your eyeballs are extremely steady and the eyelids do not flicker or fall. Try to imagine sleeping with the eyes open but with the sight fixed on the crystal. It should not wander. The mind should be steady and quiet. You will have to exert yourself to practice this daily. It is easy to learn but difficult to practise.

In the third stage, while continuing the trataka, think that you are going within yourself. Detach the mind from the act of seeing. The eyes may remain open, they may gaze at the crystal, but the mind must go inside. When the mind becomes introvert there should be no thought or desire. The mind must be dissociated from external objects. It is possible that in such a stage one may see dreams and may feel like going to sleep. The desire to sleep is sometimes so strong that the seeker feels lazy and wants to sleep. At this critical time the mind readily deceives. It brings such thoughts and advises you to go out to the lower levels of grossness. In spite of that you should continue to gaze. In this state with open eyes you may see dreams. The sadhaka sees forms in the crystal, forms which appear to be moving and active and talking. It is just what one experiences in dreams which have little relation to the waking state.

When you see forms in the crystal even while gazing at the crystal, you should gaze as if you are looking for or searching for something. Just as when we are observing something critically our minds are attuned to it, so also at this time you should create such an attitude of the mind. The look must be a searching look. If anything is seen the mind should observe it steadily and critically. By a little mental effort you will be able to see in detail every form. Try to make it mentally clear. For example, what does the form of the person observed look like? Who can he be? What is indicated on his features and what does he intend saying or doing? What has he in his hands? With whom is he talking? What does he say? Practise this daily. The first course of trataka is prescribed for six months.

Nada Yoga

THE SCIENCE OF SOUND

Nada yoga is the science of sound. The fundamental principle of nada yoga is that our world is based on one nada, that the entire universe is a system of sound principles.

Those of us who are not materialistic in outlook believe that the body is not the ultimate. It is only a gross layer. There is a body subtler than the gross one, the pranic or the vital body. You know that prana is the life-principle and has five subdivisions: *prana, apana, vyana, samana* and *udana*. This is a functional division of prana. There are still subtler subdivisions, five in number, which are also responsible for acts like sneezing, blinking, etc. These are also the actions of the same vital energy, prana. Beyond our physical body exists a mental body through which we are able to think and understand. This constitutes the mental layer of our consciousness. Subtler than this is the layer of intelligence of the astral body. This is often experienced in dreams or visions. The fifth is the subtlest layer, the layer of absolute consciousness. In yogic parlance these layers or sheaths are described as the *annamaya, pranayama, manomaya, vijnanamaya* and *anandamaya koshas*. Therefore, those who practice yoga assert that the physical body is not everything; you see it is just a starting point.

Likewise, the external sounds are not the only sounds. In our body also, there are infinite sound vibrations in the different layers of consciousness, the permutations and combinations of which go to form this body. The nada yogis say that in the beginning there was only one sound and that sound was the sacred *Om,* and that later on, through its sound vibrations, this universe came into existence. Those who have read the Bible will be familiar with the observation: "In the beginning, there was the Word". Thus there was nothing but the sound. The *Om* or cosmic sound vibrated all throughout and everywhere. These vibrations of *Om* created the first sound principle, and out of this principle emanated matter. Thus, according to the tenets of nada yoga, the entire body and the entire creation is nothing but the solidification of sound waves. This is technically called the *nada Brahman* (sound cosmos).

If you care to study the science of music, you will come to know that every sound has a form, it is not a mere vibration. The notes of music can be solidified. Every sound can be given a form – just as you see a stone, a chair, a leaf, etc. The sound can be converted into energy. This energy can again be converted into sound. The sound can be converted into an object and the object can be disintegrated into atomic particles. Those who are familiar with the theory of Einstein will bear this out.

Thus we know that in this world whatever things exist, their ultimate substance and nucleus are one, only the forms are different. All objects, though their forms are different, have a common inner substance. The nada yogis tell you are that all your constituents, which have assumed gross form, are based upon the vibration of the sound principle. This constitutes their metaphysics and philosophy.

In the science of yoga it is said that somewhere in us is a sound. It is expressed as the inner voice, the voice from heaven, the whisper from the unknown, the *akasha vani*, and, in everyday language, as the language of the soul. It is the voice of the soul, the voice of pure reason, and we should not confuse it with anything else.

In our spiritual body there is a centre from which some-one who is sitting speaks. When and with whom he speaks cannot be explained, defined or described. The practice of nada yoga makes our mind more and more subtle so that it becomes completely purified of all objective notions. It is then that we know and hear the ultimate sound.

When you start this practice, it first appears that you hear a sound like the one produced by the working of a textile mill. You close your eyes and try to listen to such a sound. Therefore, if you still try to hear the inner voice more minutely, you will hear something akin to the chirping sound of birds. Later on, you will experience the full-throated nightingale singing. But the question arises as to how to investigate the sounds.

The simplest method is to try to have a grip over the first available sound, whatever it may be, and concentrate upon it. After some time you will feel it coming closer and becoming louder, and from the background you will also experience another faint sound. It will indeed be very faint, but the moment you apprehend it, leave aside the original sound and concentrate upon the faint sound. After some time you will feel it coming closer and becoming louder in volume. After some concentration you will also experience another faint sound. As before, you have to grasp this sound and concentrate upon it till another emerges. Gradually, you will be chasing a number of sounds, one after the other.

I have only mentioned three sounds, but other sounds heard are those of the bell, flute, conch, etc. The scriptures describe ten types of sounds, beginning with the sound of a cricket, and these are supposed to be the sounds normally heard by the practitioner.

Everyone has a different experience of sounds. So, which specific type of sound is heard is not of much importance, but it is useful as indicating one's progress when practising higher sadhanas.

There are different methods of practising nada yoga. First, you practise bhramari pranayama. You have to inhale deeply and when you exhale, you produce a humming sound and concentrate upon it at the throat pit, the location of *vishuddhi chakra*. The 'zzz' sound will continue for about thirty seconds.

Here, you do not have to be mindful of sounds. In nada yoga you have to proceed mechanically till the first sound is produced. Then you have to concentrate on this sound. This constitutes the first stage.

In the second stage you have to plug your ears with the index fingers, breathe in and, as before, at the time of exhaling produce the humming sound. The teeth should be kept slightly apart. Concentrate on the sound as if it is emanating from the centre of the head.

Keep on producing the sound and then concentrate on the vibrations. Also try to investigate some other sound which is at the back of that vibration. In the first state, if you create Om vibrations, you may with a little attention discover a faint bird-like sound.

In the third stage you have to keep the ears plugged, but make no audible sound. Try to listen to the first sound, whatever its nature might be. Go on listening and feel that the sound is getting closer and louder. That is the first sound. Now, in its background you will hear another sound. It is important that the third meditation of nada yoga should be practised both with the ears plugged and without making any audible sound.

In the fourth stage, do not plug the ears or produce any sound. At about eleven in the night or at four in the morning take a bath or have a wash and sit in any comfortable posture. Try to catch the first available sound. You should feel the first sound and let it get louder. Then the second faint sound will emanate. Concentrate on it, and give up concentrating on the first sound. Let the second faint sound get louder. Again, a third faint sound will emanate. Likewise you have to go on meditating on sounds, thus discovering more and more subtle sounds.

By the practice of nada yoga the confusions of the brain are removed, the mind attains peace and meditation becomes successful.

Ajapa Japa

THE SPONTANEOUS MANTRA OF THE BREATH

The practice of ajapa is as old as the Hindu scriptures. In some of the old scriptures on yoga we find some passages and stanzas which declare that the breath goes in with the sound of *so* and comes out with the sound of *ham*. This is the sound of the *ajapa gayatri* which the *jiva* (individual soul) continuously repeats. Rishi Valmiki was initiated by Muni Narada in the technique of taking the inverted name, which is this very ajapa. Even now a number of spiritual sects in India practise ajapa. The ancient sages also practised ajapa. Mahatma Gandhi has written in his books that the 'name' should come out from within the heart and not only from the mouth. When the 'name' comes out from the mouth it is called japa. When it comes from the heart it is called ajapa.

Ajapa is a very important sadhana and through it one can have direct experience of samadhi. In order to attain samadhi in all other yogic practices one has to control and suspend the breath. The breathing system, however, remains normal in the continuous practice of ajapa, and even in samadhi there is no change.

Ajapa is a part of kriya. A Muslim saint, while referring to this ajapa, has said: "I am experiencing the fourth dimension of consciousness". Again, he has said: "This awareness of *ham* starts from the navel centre. When it comes out, it is reversed". So, you produce *ham* from the navel centre, and when it has been completely produced, you reverse it by *so*. Now it becomes *hamso*.

There are certain practices in yoga where one becomes introvert and there is an automatic suspension of the breath. The difficulty is that the aspirant becomes extrovert after a little meditation if the capacity of the lungs is not adequate, which is the case with many of us. In the practice of ajapa, however, this difficulty is solved. The ajapa practice is complete in itself. Those who have read the *Yogasutras* of Patanjali know that first of all one has to concentrate on a definite object, first with open eyes, then one must meditate with closed eyes. This is concentration on a subtle form. After that, when concentration on a subtle form is complete, one must concentrate on the simple awareness of its presence. When a schoolboy goes to the higher class he dispenses with the books of the lower class. In yoga also, one has to take up a certain practice and then give it up when success is achieved in that practice.

In the *Bhagavad Gita* also, there is a clear reference to ajapa. It says that some practices merge prana in apana. Others, apana in prana, or they merge prana in prana. Prana is the ingoing breath; apana is the outgoing breath. *So* represents prana and *ham* represents apana. Some aspirants merge prana with apana, i.e. they join *so* with *ham* which then becomes *soham*. Other aspirants join apana with prana, i.e. they join *ham* and *so*, which becomes *hamso*. There are other sadhakas who join prana with prana. This practise will be dealt with later.

In the *Gita* there is one more reference to ajapa: "Having equalized the prana and apana moving in the nasal region, let the flow of the ingoing and outgoing breaths in the nostrils be equal in length and duration."

Thus the practice of ajapa is most important and has been referred to in the scriptures. It is complete in itself and through it one can enter the spiritual realms even without the help of a spiritual master. If you merely take *soham* for ajapa, you can complete six stages in *soham* itself.

In the successful practice of trataka, one attains inner visualization of the object one meditates on. But after that the way is closed. You cannot reach the stage of samadhi all by yourself through other yogic practices. You need a spiritual master to tell you what the next practice is. In the case of ajapa, however, you do not need a guide.

It is said that one should do a japa that will never end. It must be co-extensive with infinity. Well, we do not know any such mantra. Therefore, there should be a method of repeating the mantra so that it does not end. This is achieved through the practice of ajapa japa, when the mantra is adjusted to the breathing process, thus, mantra awareness continues throughout.

Before explaining the actual practice of ajapa, let us explain one more thing. If your hand gets hurt and I ask you if you feel the pain, you will reply in the affirmative. But where is the pain? You will say it is in your mind. This is locating the pain. In yoga also, there is a process of locating consciousness.

Where is your consciousness? Think for a few minutes about where you are. You do not know where you are. Your awareness or consciousness is now extrovert and dissipated, but it can be located at any particular centre of your body.

Suppose you suddenly see a light on your mental plane while meditating. You see it for a second. In yogic language, this is called locating the consciousness. This is an important fact in the path of spiritual progress. It is through this process that the yogis transmit their consciousness.

We normally do not know where our astral body is. Through the practice of ajapa you will be able to know where your awareness is.

There are two birds, black and white, tied to a peg with two ropes. They fly for a while, but have to come back because they are tied. They fly many times. Ultimately they get tired and sleep peacefully near the peg. This illustration refers to ida and pingala. They are two birds as it were. The flow in the right nostril corresponds to pingala (sun channel) and the flow in the left nostril corresponds to ida (moon channel). The alternate functioning of ida and pingala keeps one away from one's inner consciousness. So long as they work alternately, samadhi cannot be attained. It is only when the two birds – ida and pingala – are tired and they retire to the centre, the self, that the sushumna awakens and the process of meditation becomes automatic.

According to *swara yoga,* when both the nostrils flow equally it indicates that the sushumna is flowing. At this time one should give up all worldly work and meditate. It is a common experience that sometimes the meditation is equally successful. This is because there is harmony in the entire system. When the sushumna does not function, one does not achieve concentration even with effort. So it is important that the functioning of ida and pingala should be harmonized by yoga practices and meditation, making it possible for sushumna to function.

In order to stop the chain of thoughts, one has to observe the thoughts, to see them consciously. During ajapa you must have a complete and unceasing awareness of what you are doing. Like the oilstream which does not break in the middle, let your consciousness also be continuous. Maintain continuous awareness of what you are doing.

The next important point in ajapa is that one should keep the mind fixed on the centre of meditation. It may be *ajna chakra* (the third eye or eyebrow centre) or *anahata chakra* (the heart centre) or any other centre in the body. This is called *ishwara pranidhana*. Three things are very important in ajapa: *tapasya* (sustained endurance), *swadhyaya* (continuous self-observation) and also ishwara pranidhana (fixing the mind on the centre of meditation). Yet three more important points of ajapa practice are: deep breathing, relaxation and total awareness. Not a single breath should go unnoticed. There should be no automatic breathing. You must have unceasing awareness of every ingoing and outgoing breath. As soon as the mind wanders, bring it back to the breath.

Thus ajapa is adjusting a mantra to the breathing process. It can be practised anywhere: in a chair, on the floor or in any asana, particularly padmasana, siddhasana, siddha yoni asana or sukhasana.

The most important point in ajapa japa is that firstly you have to breathe in and out consciously and not automatically. Automatic breathing goes on at night also. It is not ajapa. You must consciously notice every ingoing and outgoing breath. Like a watchman, watch the continuous and unceasing consciousness of the two breaths. You must also observe how far the breath is going in. When you breathe in, the abdomen should rise first, then chest. Breathing out, relax chest then abdomen. Lie down and feel as if you are going to sleep. You should breathe like a person who breathes deeply in sound sleep. After continued practice your breathing will be complete, systematic and proportionate. The normal rate of inhalation and exhalation is fifteen times a minute each. In one hour, nine hundred breaths and in twenty-four hours 21,600 breaths are drawn. A person who has perfected ajapa will do 21,600 rounds of japa per day.

As and when the concentration becomes deep, the breathing will become slow. Instead of fifteen rounds, you will do ten rounds a minute. In japa you make the breath as long and as deep as when you are snoring. Longevity is increased by doing so because the entire system becomes absolutely calm and steady, thereby expending less prana.

Now we come to the technical side of ajapa. There is no other technical difficulty in doing ajapa. The only difficulty is tapas, which means sustained endurance. You must sit in one posture. The body should not shake and the mind should not run here and there. It is not physical mortification. It is sustained endurance. You take the pledge that you will do ajapa for forty-five minutes every day. One day you do it, but the next day you lose patience; the third day you lose interest, and on the fourth day you lose everything. Keep up your resolve and continue with patience for a month or so, whether it is for ten minutes or one hour.

Practice note

There is misunderstanding about the *soham* mantra. *Soham* does not merely mean 'I am that'. *So* is the introspective sound of the ingoing breath, while the vibrations that are created on the outgoing breath are like *ham*. At any rate, *soham* merely indicates the complete circuit of introspection upon the two breaths. You need not think at all of the literal meaning of the word *soham*.

Outline of practice

Sit in a comfortable posture. Relax.
Start deep breathing.
Then join *so* with the ingoing breath and *ham* with the outgoing breath.
Feel that you are introspecting on *soham*.
There should be no mental pause between *so* and *ham*.
There should be continuity.
After *ham* pause a little.
Breathe in with *so*, breathe out with *ham*.
There should be continuous awareness of the ingoing and outgoing breaths and of *soham*.
After some time stop ajapa and go into *shoonya*.
Take your mind to the place in between the two eyebrows (*bhrikuti*) and concentrate on ajna chakra at the eyebrow centre.
You can also meditate on the *hridaya chakra* (heart centre) if you like.
Think of nothing. Just become blank like shoonya.
Whatever thoughts come to you, keep on removing them.
Only think of blankness.
Let this continue for a couple of minutes.
After that, again start ajapa.
In ajapa, first there will be concentration on the two streams of breath followed by the synchronizing of *soham*.
You can adjust any other mantra you like with the breathing process.

PRACTICE

Stage 1

Relax yourself physically and mentally.
Make yourself as light and relaxed as possible.
Put aside for a while all your worries and problems.
Feel calmness and serenity, peace and bliss, complete mental relaxation before you start the practice of ajapa.
Feel that you are sitting comfortably.
Begin breathing as above.
Be conscious of every ingoing and outgoing breath. The ingoing breath goes up from the navel to the throat and the outgoing breath goes down from the throat to the navel region.
No automatic breathing, but conscious, deep and relaxed breathing.
Do not produce any sound while breathing.
Feel the two streams of breath.
Intensify the awareness of prana.
Now add *soham* to this.
As the prana rises with inhalation, feel the vibration of *so*, and as the prana descends with exhalation, feel the vibrations of *ham*.
Continue to breathe in and out and try to synchronize *soham* with it.
So sounds during inhalation and the ascending of the prana in the psychic passage.
Ham sounds during exhalation and the descending of the prana in the psychic passage.
Maintain unceasing awareness of the prana and the mantra.
Now centralize your consciousness either between the eyebrows (ajna chakra) or at the heart (anahata chakra).
Stop thinking. Centralize your awareness.
Create a vacuum. Set aside all thoughts.
Simple awareness of a particular centre should be maintained.

Continue breathing consciously in and out.
Start *soham* with the ingoing and outgoing breaths as usual. Continue this practice for some time.
Practice this first stage of ajapa for a month. After you perfect it, go to the second stage.

Stage 2

During the first practice of ajapa you introspected on *so* with the ingoing breath and *ham* with the outgoing breath. Now, in the second practice, reverse the whole emphasis of the process.
Introspect on *ham* while exhaling and *so* while inhaling. *Ham* is the introspective sound vibration of the outgoing prana as it descends in the psychic passage. *So* is the introspective sound vibration of the ingoing prana as it ascends in the psychic passage.
There should be no pause between *hamso* throughout. After the ajapa of *hamso*, become blank. Do not think of anything. Take your consciousness either to ajna chakra or anahata chakra.
There should be total awareness of the centre of meditation. Do not put any pressure on the centre, simply concentrate your mind there.
The process of deep breathing, relaxation, total awareness and so on will be the same in this second practice of *hamso* as in the practice of *soham*.
One may practise this *hamso* for a month. After achieving success in it, turn to the third stage.

Stage 3

In the first practice of ajapa, you formulated your consciousness in the pattern of *soham*.
In the second practice you reversed it to *hamso*.
Now we come to the third practice.
Relax yourself mentally.
The relaxation can be achieved successfully by autosuggestion and by awaking awareness of 'I am'.

If one has tensions there is another method of relaxation through counting.
Count one with the ingoing breath.
Count one with the outgoing breath.
Count two with ingoing breath.
Count two with the outgoing breath.
Go on counting like this until four.
When you come to five be alert.
Try to maintain undistracted awareness.
Feel that you are definitely counting five. Say mentally, 'I am aware of five with the ingoing breath and I am aware of five with the outgoing breath.' Then go on counting till nine. Again, when you come to ten, be alert.
Maintain fullest awareness that you are counting ten.
Repeat this whole process a couple of times.
Now start rhythmic and deep breathing.
Absolutely peaceful, prolonged and relaxed breathing.
Practise mindfulness all throughout the process of breathing.
Introspect neither on *soham* nor upon *hamso*, but with the ingoing breath upon the individual *so*, and with outgoing breath on the individual *ham*. Do not be aware of either *soham* or *hamso*.
Just feel *so* with inhalation and the upward movement of consciousness in the psychic passage, and *ham* with exhalation and the downward movement in the psychic passage.
Individual *so* and individual *ham*.
When this practice is over, create a mental vacuum.
Localize your consciousness at any centre of meditation.
Again start breathing consciously and continue the practice of individual *so* and individual *ham* for a month or so.

Stage 4

Close your eyes and sit in a steady posture.
Mentally relax yourself by auto-suggestion, awareness of self, by the feeling of peace, happiness and bliss.

Start rhythmic breathing.
Breathe in and out from the navel.
Be aware of the different centres through which your breath passes, right from the nose to navel, and from navel to nose.
Rhythmic, peaceful and relaxed breathing.
Now, *so* with the ingoing breath and *ham* with the outgoing breath. But the form of your consciousness will be a continuity of *sohamso*.
So merging in *ham* and *ham* merging in *so*, making an endless circle.
Prolong the vibrations of *ham* and join them with the vibration of the ingoing *so*.
Prolong the vibrations of *so* and join them with *ham*.
The latter part of *ham* joins the early part of *so* and becomes a continuous circle of *sohamso*.
Now stop this practice and empty your mind.
Create blankness.
Focus your consciousness on any of the centres of meditation.
Remove all thoughts.
Again after some time start the endless circle of *soham-soham*.
At the end of a practice of half an hour or an hour, heighten your imagination of peace and rest. Feel mentally, 'There is happiness and peace.'
All these practices of ajapa are mental, not verbal.

Introduction to Stage 5

Thus far, four practices of ajapa have been explained. Now we go on to the fifth stage which is rather more difficult and commands greater imagination on the part of the aspirant. It consists of rotating the consciousness within the spinal column.

The process of concentration and meditation consists of two factors: control of the external consciousness and expression of the calm and quiet soul in us.

A burning lamp cannot radiate its full illumination if its glass is covered with soot. It is only when the glass is cleaned that the lamp shines most brightly. Similarly, the light or the power of the soul is within us, but it does not manifest itself in our daily lives because of the hindrance of thinking principles, the vagaries of the mind, dissipations and distractions. Meditation helps one to annihilate the sense consciousness and awaken self-awareness. It removes the impurities of the mind.

There are different systems of meditation. The first meditation belongs to the group of the body; the second meditation belongs to the group of the mind, i.e. thinking of an idea; the third meditation belongs to the group of the intellect; and the fourth process of meditation belongs to the higher region.

Light manifests itself when the physical consciousness, the mental consciousness, the intellectual awareness, and lastly the personality itself, when all these are transcended in toto. So long as you do not transcend the body, the mind and the intellect, you will not attain perfect serenity and peace. The various practices of ajapa aim to achieve this.

In an academic career one has to go through primary, higher secondary, college and university education in order to get the highest degree. Similarly in meditation there are four stages. First is relaxation, second is awareness, third is unification, and the fourth is forgetfulness. This has been explained in the previous practices of ajapa.

Now we come to the fifth stage of ajapa. The first important thing in ajapa is rhythmic breathing. The second important thing is mindfulness. All through the process of meditation you must be mindful of every activity you do. If, while practising meditation, you forget that you are meditating you will never gain success in meditation.

While meditating there comes a state of unmindfulness akin to sleep, and this is the trouble with almost every aspirant who meditates. You keep on thinking of a certain problem for fifteen minutes or so. During this period, when you were brooding over the problem, you were not mindful that you were brooding. It is only when you finish the process of brooding that you realize that you were thinking about such a thing. This is not meditation.

In meditation, whatever practice you are following you should be mindful. Therefore, we always emphasize one point: be aware of what you are doing. Be conscious that you are counting. Be mindful that you are visualizing, breathing – in short, be absolutely awake and vigilant. You have to be conscious of every process of breathing, and mindfulness should have an unceasing continuity.

During meditation practice, if you count one, two, three, your mind should not be unaware for even a single second. Even if it wanders, let it, but be aware that it is wandering. If you concentrate, be aware that you are concentrating. It is the very nature of the mind to wander and sleep. You need not worry about this, but be fully aware of every tendency of the mind.

Whenever your mind, your consciousness, your awareness dissipates, be alert. No mental activity should go unnoticed. You should never be unmindful of the processes of concentration. This is the fundamental and the only point to be remembered. If you fail to remember and understand this most important point, you will never achieve success in meditation even if you meditate for a century.

Second is rhythmic breathing through the psychic passage, and mindfulness.

Third is rotation of the vibration of *so* and *ham* through the psychic passage.

It is a psychological fact that when you want to control the mind it wanders ruthlessly and you fail to control it. But if you quietly watch the mental activity, it will stop. Therefore, in all the four practices of ajapa we have tried to emphasize this truth that, instead of commanding the mind to stop forcibly, you should be mindful of its every activity.

You have been given the practice of rhythmic breathing, mindfulness, synchronization of mantra with the ingoing and outgoing breaths, and finally of creating temporary blankness in the mind.

In the fifth stage of ajapa you have to use a lot of imagination in the beginning. Later on it will become a real process. In the previous practices you introspected with the inhalation moving up from the navel and with the exhalation moving down to the navel. Now you have to change this process and circulate your consciousness in the spinal column through the six psychic centres.

The six chakras or psychic centres, starting from the bottom, are: *mooladhara*, between the anus and the genitals at the perineum in males and at the cervix in females; *swadhisthana*, at the base of the spine; *manipura*, at the level of the navel in the spine; *anahata*, at the level of the heart in the spine; *vishuddhi*, at the level of the throat in the spine and *ajna*, in the centre of the head at the top of the spine. First relax yourself mentally and physically, and sit in a comfortable posture.

Stage 5

Take to rhythmic and prolonged breathing.

Be mindful throughout.

Now, exhaling take the breath to ajna chakra, then to vishuddhi chakra, anahata chakra, manipura chakra, swadhisthana chakra and lastly to mooladhara chakra.

Circulate the breath-consciousness from ajna chakra to mooladhara chakra through the spinal passage.

Now maintain your consciousness at mooladhara chakra for a while.

Locate the inverted triangle and within it, the *kundalini*.

Kundalini is the dormant potentiality in us which sleeps like a snake coiled at the base of the spinal column.

In the framework of the triangle is the kundalini, coiled three and half times around a lingam.

Meditate on this kundalini for a few seconds.

Now, inhale from mooladhara through the spinal column and the six chakras, then exhale down.

After simple rotation of the breathing consciousness in the spinal column, add *so* and *ham* to the inhalation and exhalation respectively.

The passage of consciousness will be the spinal column, and the centre of consciousness will be the mooladhara triangle and the kundalini within it.

Say *so* while breathing in.

Take the vibration of *so* up to ajna chakra with inhalation.

From ajna chakra through the spinal column descend to mooladhara chakra with the mental vibration of *ham*.

Retain the breath-consciousness there for a while.

Meditate on the kundalini.

Now, with the vibration of *so* you ascend the spinal passage.

The ascending passage is from mooladhara chakra to ajna chakra with *so*, and the descending passage is from ajna chakra to mooladhara chakra with *ham*.

Descend the spinal passage with *ham* and then take some rest.

Just be aware of yourself, do not create blankness.

To sum up, with the vibration of *so* you ascend in the spinal column, then descend to mooladhara with *ham*.

There you retain the breath outside and locate the kundalini for a few seconds.

Then you ascend the spinal column with the vibration of *so* and you exhale with *ham*.

After exhalation, rest and practise simple self-awareness.

Thus, the fifth practice of ajapa consists of rotating the consciousness in the ascending and descending passage of the spinal column with the vibration of *so* and *ham*.

Summary

First is relaxation.

Second is rhythmic breathing through the spinal passage and mindfulness.

Third is rotation of the vibrations of *so* and *ham* though the spinal passage.

Fourth is retention in mooladhara chakra and meditation on the inverted triangle and the serpent power encased within it.

Be constantly aware of the ascending consciousness, locating or centralizing the consciousness and of descending consciousness.

When exhaling, it is called 'descending consciousness'.

When you meditate on mooladhara chakra, it is locating or centralizing the consciousness.

When you inhale, it is called 'ascending consciousness'.

In this practice of ajapa, the important things to be considered are rhythmic breathing, heightened imagination, perfect and continuous mindfulness, complete relaxation and awareness of what you are doing.

The best method of mental relaxation is self-awareness and auto-suggestion.

Rotating the consciousness seems to be a little difficult in the beginning because it requires great imagination, but with a little practice, it later becomes quite real and easy.

This practice is very important because if one can do it successfully, one will have peace, serenity, good dreams and a change in mental outlook. It is said that the person whose kundalini awakens gains peace first and knowledge next. This meditation should be considered successful if the practitioner gains peace and wisdom.

This being over, we come to the last stage.

Stage 6

This practice is more difficult and requires greater imagination, patience and control of the breathing process.

Loosen your clothes.

Sit straight with your spinal column erect.

Interlock your hands and keep them on your lap or on your knees.

Set aside all your mental tensions and worries.

Practise self-awareness.

Use auto-suggestion. Imagine peace and joy, and relax yourself completely.
Now with your thumbs, plug your ears.
Close your eyes and lips with your fingers.
Begin deep breathing.
After you have taken the breath in, close your nostrils with the middle fingers of each hand.
Then rotate your consciousness in the spinal column.
With the vibrations of *so*, ascend from mooladhara chakra to ajna chakra.
With the vibrations of *ham*, descend from ajna chakra to mooladhara chakra.
Then release the breath and take a little rest.
During this period of rest, practise self-awareness and mindfulness.
In the second phase of the sixth stage of ajapa, you need not close your eyes, ears, mouth and nose.
Simply breathe in.
Retain.
During the period of retention, rotate your consciousness in the spinal column, from ajna chakra to mooladhara chakra.
Stay at mooladhara chakra for a while.
Now ascend, and then exhale.
Take rest and practise self-awareness.

Conclusion

The exposition of the method of ajapa japa being practical, not much has been said here of the psychological significance of this practice. It is, however, not to be forgotten that ajapa japa offers significant benefits for mental disorders and its therapeutic effects can hardly be over-emphasized.

Ajapa japa has also a sacred significance which has been hinted at in several cryptic and mystic formula in ancient literature. This was a secret treasure jealously guarded through the centuries and was told only to deserving and earnest aspirants.

Yoga Nidra

PSYCHIC SLEEP

The simple and useful practice of the art of sleeping which the yogis know, if explained with certain modifications, can prove infinitely beneficial to many people. It may be called psychic sleep.

Very few people know how to sleep. People often go to sleep while thinking or reading. During the act of thinking, they do not know when sleep comes. To fall asleep with a mind entangled in thoughts is not beneficial to health and mind. It is not good to sleep with a mind full of anxiety and disturbances. This sleep does not provide full rest to the body. Tiredness is not cast off completely. One has bad dreams, digestion is not perfect and on the following morning one does not feel energetic and pleasant. To sleep thus is unhealthy and unscientific.

You may have doubts as to what particular thing there can possibly be in the act of sleeping which needs to be learned. Sleep comes to everybody. It is quite natural for everybody to have sleep. There is nothing particular, of course, to be learned. But you will see and realize that sleep is an important thing in our life. The effect of sleep influences our mind, activities, nature, character and intelligence.

Let us take an example. If you make a habit of getting up early in the morning and give it a strictly practical shape in your everyday life, you will find that there will be a thorough change in your life. Its effect will be on all matters connected with your living. Firstly, you will feel energetic, strong and refreshed. If you had been complaining of want of time, you would now find that the day is too long and you have not so much work. Not for a day or two only, but if you make this a life-long routine, you will feel this. You will always have perfect health. You will not have a feeling of exhaustion after any hard work. There will never be a complaint about sleeplessness (insomnia). The mind will always remain cheerful and peaceful. You will be endowed with the greatest success in all activities of life. The condition is that you must be strict in following this routine. Then only you will see the result. This and this one routine only will be able to awaken all potentialities latent in you. You will be master of extraordinary willpower.

Everybody takes sleep to be just a simple and natural affair without any importance, and it will be no exaggeration to say that no worldly man knows the scientific way of sleeping. No householder knows how to sleep. Householders have to work hard. If they learn the process of psychic sleep they will have extraordinary benefits. They will complete their sleep and derive maximum advantage with minimum hours of sleep.

In general, people experience a feeling of tiredness of body and heaviness of head after leaving their bed in the morning. Some people experience feelings of lethargy when they wake up. They do not feel like getting out of bed and they keep on dozing in a half awake state. There are many who sleep for eight long hours or even more, but feel as if they have not completed their sleep. For an average healthy person, eight hours of sleep is not only quite sufficient but is rather more than the actual requirement. Many people do not get sleep unless they take bromide or other tranquillizers. Thus we see that while many people suffer from excessive sleep, there is quite a large number of those who do not get sleep at all. Others get no sleep unless they read some books or novels. This habit is also bad for health. By reading in a lying posture the eyes are subjected to undue pressure with the result that they get tired and exhausted due to excessive strain, and sleep comes with this induced lethargy in the organs. This is a bad way of going to sleep. There are other people who do not get to sleep without having a massage. This habit is not only bad but is dangerous for those who are rheumatic. If this facility is not available when one is away from home, one does not sleep. These are all bad habits and we should take them to be ailments of sleep. Sleep should be natural and should come in a proper and natural way.

There is one more problem. A man of the present age remains tremendously busy. In the modern industrial and material world, an average man keeps running after high aims and desires. We know of the busy life of people in the big cities. There are some people who are so very busy in multifarious activities that they do not get time to sleep properly or to take proper rest. This is a problem for them. Businessmen, doctors, social workers, government or other officers, all have some difficulty regarding sleep. There is one golden rule which can be prescribed for all such people by which they can complete their requirements of sleep by lying in bed for only three hours. With this short interval of sleep they can get rid of their exhaustion caused by twenty-one hours of hard work. Napoleon is said to be one of those who slept a minimum of hours. It is said that he had to stay on horseback for days together and he completed his sleep even in the saddle. Gandhiji was also a light sleeper, he slept easily while travelling to and from programs. His hard and continuous brainwork is known to all. What were the reasons for their success? They were yogis in a true sense. They possessed full concentration of mind. They were busy after fulfilment of their goals with deep concentration. Concentration has tremendous powers. It is said that yogis never sleep. They always keep their minds towards their goal with undiverted attention. A yogi transforms his sleep into samadhi.

Just as the body rests while sleeping, the mind should also get a similar rest. Even during the night, the running of the mind does not cease. When we fall into sleep with multifarious thoughts, some thoughts (involving passion, greed, pride, attachment and all sorts of things) appear in different shapes and forms. When the mind wanders about here and there, one does not have sleep and is engrossed in horrible dreams. The mind is not peaceful and there is no feeling of being refreshed. Passionate thoughts based on fictitious events appear even at the dead of night and cause the soul to wander and get tired. These undesirable thoughts need to be diverted. If the mind is taken away from all these feelings and is turned towards one particular direction, one can attain peace and pleasure of mind.

Sleep is a lower stage of samadhi. While sleeping, man forgets all worldly troubles, anxieties, tiresome feelings and he travels into another world; no amount of abuse will affect or enrage him. In samadhi, also, man is away from all the feelings and sensations relating to this world; the organs do not communicate any feeling. But there is a difference between sleep and samadhi. In sleep one has neither knowledge of, nor power to control, oneself. In samadhi, although the organs do not communicate to him ideas connected with this world, one is quite within one's soul and has full knowledge of everything, but that is a very high stage, rather the highest, when the self is in a state of complete knowledge and infinite light. And then this world appears to be completely dark.

Generally, some people suffer from sleeplessness in varying degrees and others suffer from excessive sleep. If we think over this with a cool and pure mind, we shall realize how many long and precious hours we lose and spoil by sleeping uselessly. If we had used this costly time in doing some important work we should have achieved marvellous results.

In a nutshell, if we sleep just for the necessary hours and use the rest of our time in constructive work relating to our own life or that of others, we can attain a high position in society. All the time that we spend in useless sleep can better be utilized for study, earning money, in service of people or in spiritual practices for attaining self-realization.

When just a little sleep can suffice, where is the necessity of long sleep? It is necessary for all of us to know something about the science of sleeping. What should be the quality of sleep? How many hours should we sleep? How should we sleep? How can we get rid of our feelings of tiredness quickly? How can mental tensions be diverted? What sort of sleep will bring us freshness and energy? Practical processes relating to sleep will be explained here along with a few necessary rules for efficient sleeping. For example, excessive sleep indicates inertia and sleeplessness is the result of mental tensions. Both are undesirable.

It is good to avoid sleeping with diffused thoughts. As all daily duties are properly attended to and are given due importance, similarly the act of sleeping should also be treated in the same way. The mind should be given this training. A machine which works throughout the day without interruption gets heated. Sleep is a cooling device. It recharges the battery of our body which gets discharged while functioning during the day. Energy that we spend in hard toil is recouped. Before lying down for sleep, sit for a while on the bed calmly and quietly, say for two to four minutes. Shake from your mind all thoughts about the activities of the day. A simple way of doing this is a to start mental japa or ishta mantra. Any disturbing thoughts of the day will automatically be driven away. Then meditate on your ishta (desired deity) for sometime and lie down in bed in this state.

Yoga nidra is a more efficient and effective form of psychic and physiological rest and rejuvenation than conventional sleep. However, through yoga nidra, we are not only relaxing, but restructuring and reforming our whole personality from within. Release of tension, relaxation and peace of mind are the secrets of transformation. When a man is under tension, his behaviour is influenced, and when he relaxes, he becomes natural. If you practise yoga nidra, then the nature of your mind can be changed, diseases can be cured and your creative genius can be restored. Subconscious and unconscious mind are the most powerful forces in the human being. This simple practice of yoga nidra has the capacity of penetration into the depths of the human mind. Whether people have any physical, mental or emotional problems or not, yoga nidra should be practised daily to dive deep into the mind and aid in the evolution of your consciousness.

Practice 1

Please get ready for yoga nidra.

Lie down on your back on the floor in shavasana.

Keep the feet a little apart, hands by your sides with the palms turned upwards.

Close your eyes and keep them closed throughout the whole practice.

Now bring about a feeling of inner relaxation in the whole body...concentrate on the body and become aware of the importance of complete stillness. *(pause)* Develop your awareness of the body from the top of the head to the tips of the toes. Complete stillness and complete awareness of the whole body.

Continue your awareness of the whole body...the whole body... the whole body.

Mentally say to yourself: 'I am aware...I am going to practise yoga nidra...I will not sleep (unless you are practising for insomnia)...I will remain awake throughout the whole practice'. *(pause)*

Now begin to rotate your awareness throughout your whole physical body.

Repeat the different parts of the body in your mind and simultaneously become aware of that part of the body.

You can also visualize that part of the body in your mind, but don't concentrate too hard.

Right side

Become aware of the right hand. *(pause)*

Right hand thumb, second finger, third finger, fourth finger, fifth finger, palm, back of the hand, wrist, lower arm, elbow, upper arm, shoulder, armpit, right side of the waist, right hip, right thigh, knee, calf muscle, ankle, heel, sole, right big toe, second toe, third toe, fourth toe, fifth toe...

Left side

Become aware of the left hand thumb, second finger, third finger, fourth finger, fifth finger, palm, back of the hand, wrist, lower arm, elbow, upper arm, shoulder, armpit, left side of the waist, left hip, left thigh, knee, calf muscle, ankle, heel, sole, left big toe, second toe, third toe, fourth toe, fifth toe...

Back

Now come to the back. Become aware of the right buttock, left buttock, small of the back, right side of the back, left side of the back, centre of the back...right shoulderblade, left shoulderblade...centre of the shoulderblades...become aware of the spine from top to bottom...the whole back together...back of the neck, back of the head...

Front

Now go to the top of the head, the top of the head, forehead, both sides of the head, right eyebrow, left eyebrow, eyebrow centre, right eyelid, left eyelid, the right eye, the left eye, right ear, left ear, right cheek, left cheek, nose, tip of the nose, upper lip, lower lip, chin, throat, right side of the chest, left side of the chest, centre of the chest, stomach, navel, abdomen...

Major parts

The whole right leg...the whole left leg...both legs together. *(pause)*

The whole right arm...the whole left arm...both arms together. *(pause)*

The whole of the back, buttocks, spine, shoulder-blades... the whole of the front, abdomen, chest...the whole of the back and front...together...the whole of the head...the whole body together...the whole body together...the whole body together.

(Repeat one or two rounds gradually decreasing speed.)

Please do not sleep...total awareness...no sleeping...no movement. *(pause)* The whole body on the floor...become aware of your body lying on the floor. *(pause)* Your body is lying on the floor, see your body lying perfectly still on the floor...in this room. Visualize this image in your mind. Develop awareness of your physical body lying on the floor. Awareness of your physical body from top to toe. Awareness of the room and your surroundings. Start moving your body and stretching yourself. When you are wide awake, sit up slowly and open your eyes. The practice of yoga nidra is now complete.

Practice 2

Follow practice 1, relaxing and rotating the awareness around individual or major body parts, depending on time available.

Then become aware of your natural breath.

Just be aware that you are breathing in and breathing out, breathing in and breathing out. *(pause)*

Don't force the breath, just be aware of your natural breath.

Become aware of its rhythm – whether it's fast or slow, shallow or deep, but do not change it.

Only awareness.

Now begin to count mentally each respiration; inhalation and exhalation count mentally *one*, inhalation and exhalation, *two*, etc.

Count up to 27, 49, or 99, depending on the time available.

Be aware of each breath and number; if you miss one breath then you should start again.

Try to stay awake and aware as this practice likely to send you to sleep.

Therefore it is good for insomniacs.

Practice 3

Follow practice 1 and 2.
Become aware of your eyebrow centre, *bhrumadhya*.
Try and concentrate your mind on this point.
Then begin mental japa of *om* or *soham* at this point.
Continue for as long as possible; if the mind wanders, then gently bring it back to the eyebrow centre and mantra.

Practice 4

Follow practice 1. Then become aware of your natural breath for a few minutes.
Now add *om* or *soham* to the breath.
While breathing in chant mentally *om* or *soham* and repeat this mantra while breathing out.
Continue for as long as time is available.
This japa can also be done with four mantras as in *chaturtha pranayama*. That is, the mantra is chanted four times with each inhalation and each exhalation.
By doing japa in this way, the mind will become very concentrated.

Conclusion

The practice of yoga nidra can be done any time. In the midst of hard work during the day, if we get an opportunity, we should take a rest by doing this practice. Excessively busy people who do not get even ten to fifteen minutes for rest during the day, can practice yoga nidra seated in a chair in the midst of work.

Practise this sitting in a chair in the office for two or five minutes and all your feelings of tiredness and exhaustion will go. All body and mental tensions will vanish. The consumed energy of the body will be recouped to a great extent. Those who have to do a lot of brainwork are advised to do this kriya for even two minutes, several times a day.

All processes of this practice can be adjusted according to the time available. If the time available is very short, this practice should also be of short duration. If there is enough time, every part of each limb should be given sufficient time. One thing is most important: if you practise this during the day, you should be alert so that sleep does not come because this practice readily induces sleep.

There is another interesting point in this practice. If you have decided beforehand on the duration of sleep you want, you will get a mild jolt at that particular time and you will be awakened. These are facts based on years of practical experience.

What is required is that you should select one method according to your own choice and practise it continuously for some days or months. With slight alterations, these practices can grant the seeker entrance into the deeper world. You can learn practices from a guru himself. These deeper and finer practices can never be even understood without the blessing of a guru.

Antar Mouna

INNER SILENCE

When you concentrate and try to unify the vagrant tendencies of your mind, sometimes you feel strain. Because of that strain, you get a headache or some other complaint. Therefore, while practising concentration, you have to evolve a method in which there will be no strain. Just as a tired person goes to bed, falls asleep and has no struggle to get to sleep, even so there are various methods of achieving spontaneous concentration and meditation.

The best method of concentration starts with prayer. When we start concentration directly and abruptly, the influx of blood to the brain increases abruptly. Various ideas keep on haunting the mind and hamper meditation. All the impressions of actions done during the day come rushing up to the surface of the mind. If you want to meditate on *om*, you naturally desire that nothing else except *om* should come to your mind. But for various reasons your daily experiences and impressions come to you during meditation. Therefore, the time for meditation is in the early hours of the morning.

At night when drowsiness overpowers you, if you meditate on your personal deity you will succeed immensely. But the best time for meditation is in the morning between four and six.

Some people meditate at odd hours of the day. This is no doubt good but you must have experienced that by practising concentration during these hours, there is some tension felt in the brain. In fact, meditation should be spontaneous. It should be an effortless evolvement. If you practise the right technique from the very beginning you will have no difficulty.

Therefore, the first practice to bring about this state is inner silence. Inner silence has many graduated stages. In the beginning you are not to fight with your thoughts but to maintain an impartial attitude. If thoughts come to your mind let them do so. With closed eyes remain a witness of the various thoughts coming into your mind and do not try consciously to control the thought processes.

Do not be disturbed when various thoughts overwhelm you. Nor should you try to trim or eliminate those thoughts. Just close your eyes and becomes a witness. Feel as if the thoughts are passing before you gradually like a goods train.

Preparation to stage 1

The centre of meditation is the brain. If there is more or less flow of blood in the brain then meditation will not be possible. It is not possible to point out what the right proportion of circulation should be to create congenial meditation conditions. There is no instrument to point this out, but the saints have found a clue. When our thoughts assume the shape of dreams and visions float, then the brain is regarded as being in the ideal condition for meditation. As long as your thoughts do not materialize or assume forms, you are not regarded as ready for concentration and you may not be able to meditate easily.

Now let us examine actually how to practise this and what your attitude should be at that time.

Preparatory practice

Close your eyes and try to relax yourself mentally. The technique is to feel that you are going to take rest. Do not entertain any strenuous thoughts in your mind as you generally do.

Experience peace and a feeling of joy, rest and comfort.
The more you are able to relax, the more you will be able to practise concentration.
In this relaxation, try to feel that you are sitting on a chair and that your body is resting on it.
This means that you should be aware of yourself and of your position.
This is called self-awareness.
Your limbs should also relax. This may take some time.
Relaxation is a process which is strenuous in the beginning but peaceful afterwards.
Try to visualize the darkness in the forehead region behind the closed eyes.
Is the darkness changing its colour or not?
Do you see a star or anything else?
What do you see?
Some see stars, some see lights, some see a glare, some see only darkness.
Never mind whether you see anything or not. Just keep on concentrating on whatever is before you.
Many thoughts will arise. Let them.
There may be thoughts, sounds sensation or any other different feelings.
You may experience an itching sensation in your body or a tremor in your system.
Try to be a mere witness to all that.
Do not identify yourself with any sound, sensation or thought that arises in your mind.
When this is over then you should begin the actual practice of inner silence.

Introduction to stage 1

This is the first practice in inner silence. This practice evolves a technique which operates subjectively and brings about a cessation in the process of thinking. In the case of impure thoughts, awaken an awareness that you are only witnessing them while they are passing through your mental plane. If you do not identify with such thoughts, they will be suspended without any effort. You should not be disturbed by them. You should not feel elated by good thoughts and think that your meditation is very nice just because good thoughts alone come to you. Thoughts of any type, shade and dimension, whether good or bad, should merely be observed without any involvement.

During the process of witnessing your thoughts, sometimes there comes a of state of mental suspension and for a moment we forget that we were witnessing our thoughts. Then confusion occurs in the realm of awareness. We do not know what we are doing. Later on we realize we were practising inner silence. Then we restart the practice. Again and again this suspension follows. The only way to remove this confusion in awareness is to keep on with the practice of inner silence. By practising continuously for a few days, inner silence becomes clear and ultimately the last stage of 'seeing the thoughts' is achieved.

After a successful round of practice, thoughts will not remain as gross ideas, but will appear in their astral forms as visions. Every thought will then become an astral reality with subtle dimensions.

Inner silence starts with relaxation as the first practice. Secondly, you have to become as impartial seer of your thoughts. Thirdly, do not be disturbed by any thought that comes to your mind, whether good or bad. Finally, whenever thoughts come to you in their astral forms, take it that your practice is complete.

You will be able to see your thoughts by constant practice of inner silence. But this is not to be regarded as concentration. This is only a preparatory exercise before commencing actual concentration. After achieving this state of experience you should start meditation on your desired or personal deity. You will find it is very easy to have a clear vision of the astral forms of your desired deity. You can continue your meditation on your desired deity for as long as you want.

Stage 1: Thought introspection

Before beginning the practice, you should first of all relax yourself mentally.

Sit in any comfortable asana.

Remember, in whatever posture you use, the spinal column must be kept straight.

Then relax yourself mentally.

Imagine how relaxed you feel when you come back from a hectic business round in the scorching sun and relax on a sofa in an air-conditioned room.

Be aware of this kind of relaxation.

This is preparatory to meditation.

Relaxation is an aid to concentrate, so also is auto-suggestion. Feel that you do not have to do anything and that you are experiencing joy. Thus try to relax yourself mentally.

During this stage of inner silence you should be aware that you are thinking.

'I am thinking' – this must kept in mind constantly.

The only caution is that you should not identify yourself with the thoughts.

The awareness of the thinking process should be maintained throughout.

'I am thinking' should be the constant awareness.

Introduction to Stage 2

Many thoughts arise in the mind. Sometimes they arise with compelling force and it seems as if some unseen force within us is compelling their upsurge. We may be averse to certain thoughts of passion; we may not like to enter into worries and brooding, but despite all sincere efforts we fail to check the waves.

This is a proof that we lack control over the mind and that we must evolve some effective method for settling these vagrant forces in their proper place.

If this is not done in time, then the mind will reach its breaking point and as a result, sedatives, hypnotics and narcotics will have to be introduced to ease the mental tension.

If thought waves are not regulated in time, they become part of our habit and under their hypnotic lullaby we spend, nay waste, years upon years. We only rise to the critical situation when every possibility has gone beyond our hands.

We wake up at the instance of a nervous breakdown, mental fever, neurosis and the like. It becomes too late for us to overcome them. It is beyond the power of any physician.

If care is taken well before the crisis takes place, and thought-regulation is rendered as a part of our mental habit, then we can keep away various mental ailments successfully.

What is the remedy then? Yoga has prescribed a method by which a person can, with practice, become the master of his thoughts. He need not control his thoughts. He need not kill his mind. He must only attain complete mastery over his thoughts. He who has attained mastery over his mind keeps it as his trained servant. When the mind is properly kept under control it can help you in many ways. One of the methods to train the mind is by following the second practice in the art of inner silence.

This practice of inner silence consists of creating a particular thought, voluntarily dwelling on it for some time, then rejecting it altogether.

Here you voluntarily create any thought of your liking and, after thinking it over for some minutes, you set it aside by your willpower.

It is better if you start with lower thoughts. That is to say, you should voluntarily create and dwell on themes of jealousy, anger, greed, and the like, and finally set them aside with a mental strike. We suggest such thoughts because the mind is very much accustomed to revolving around gross thoughts and, in fact, lower thoughts act as various centres of gravity to our consciousness. Pious thoughts are soon forgotten and the mind finds it easy to slip away from good thoughts, while it is almost a task to detach its interest from lower thoughts. Thoughts of jealousy, anger, greed, fear, emotion, passion and pride – all these seem to have greater affinity with the mind, while peace, compassion, love, forgiveness and so on are usually missed by the mind during meditation. Good resolves are always forgotten while evil intentions stay on.

You should therefore practise in this way: pose a particular thought, retain the same thought for some time with vivid imagination, then dispose of it. If you practise this method for some time you will learn the technique of removing any permanent thought that haunts your mind. This method of inner silence is extremely useful. Along with this, when this stage of inner silence is over, you have to meditate on your desired deity. We have already said that it is possible to have the inner vision of the deity you worship only if you have attained that proper state of concentration and realization.

Stage 2: Thought regulation

Now you have to practise inner silence.

Pose any thought. Retain it for some time.

Dash it off.

Go on doing it.

Choose your thought if you want to, but use caution; do not become one with your thoughts.

Be conscious throughout of what you are doing.

Don't let any thought come that is not willed.

Reject any thoughts that come to you of their own accord.

You should pose a thought at will. Retain it and then dash it off.

Do not get attached to the thought.

Practise with detachment.

Vividly imagine what you are thinking.

Sometimes while thinking there will be confusion.

You will not be able to say what you are thinking.

When this happens you must at once meditate on your desired deity.

Keep in view a few important points for meditation of the desired deity.
Try to think of the particular deity through general observances. Think of the whole picture of your deity.
Think of the where the deity is, and the surroundings.
Vividly imagine all this from a general image to the details.

Practical problems

Before we discuss the third stage of this practice, we will discuss a few practical problems which occur during the process of relaxation and inner silence.

The main problem is sleep which is experienced when you relax. First drowsiness dawns, then deep slumber. For those who want to remove hypertension sleep is necessary, but those who seek spiritual evolution will have to find a remedy for the trouble. If you want to attain samadhi and spiritual enlightenment, or want to contact the astral body, or the mysterious kundalini, or practise other forms of meditation, it becomes all the more essential to know the technique to overcome this difficulty. The complaint of all aspirants is that when they succeed in achieving inner silence, they fall asleep and realize it only afterwards when awareness returns. No doubt they feel fresh but spiritual evolution is arrested. Even in the case of earnest aspirants, spiritual progress is arrested because they fall asleep. Householders, who have to discharge various duties, who are always busy and under continuous strain, naturally fall asleep after even a little concentration.

But there is another difficulty, that is, if the consciousness is not partially asleep, inner silence is difficult to achieve. The mind has to be drowsy to some degree and at the same time one has to be careful not to fall asleep. Therefore, it is necessary that those who want to avoid sleep during meditation bear in mind just a few points.

First you will have to practise detachment. You will have to reject that continuity of thought by constant and persistent practice. This is one solution. The second solution is to practise pranayama when you start to fall asleep. Practise any pranayama with kumbhaka in the ratio 1:4:2. Do it three or four times, then practise concentration. This is for those who face waves of depression due to hypertension and continuous thinking. If you minimize the degree of depression, you will be able to visualize the object of your meditation very clearly.

Some people sit in padmasana and meditate for hours at a stretch and feel themselves in samadhi. But this is not samadhi. This is an after-effect of the strain of everyday life. You can, of course, remove your mental depression by this suspension, but you cannot go any further on the spiritual path. You can also practise some asanas, such as sarvangasana or sirshasana. Through asanas we can check the causes responsible for sleep. Get out of bed, take a wash and sit in any asana. Then there will be no suspension.

Some aspirants sit for meditation but do not know what they are doing. Others, having heard about the kundalini, desire to awaken it and apply extra pressure, but there is bound to be depression. Therefore, in order to avoid sleep during meditation, a light dinner, asanas and pranayama will help you best.

When you meditate with closed eyes and visions begin to appear, then there is temporary suspension of awareness. Again visions, then suspension, and once again visions. All this happens because *samskaras* float on the mental surface.

You forget so many unwanted things. You reject them and, therefore, they go into the background. In due course this brings about bad after-effects. Either rationalize your problems or sublimate them by total detachment. Your dislike for a person does not at all mean that he has gone out of your mind. On the contrary, he is very much in your mind. His memory will disturb you in meditation. So whatever difficulties we have, we should annihilate their impressions either by rationalization or by sublimation with detachment. This is another factor responsible for sleep and visions in the initial stages of meditation. The only solution to this problem is to render the mind free from day-to-day tensions by various asanas, pranayama, antar mouna, yoga nidra and meditation. Sleep is no doubt good, also the expression of astral contents in the form of visions. But as the seeking is for higher attainments, we will have to go beyond all forms of relaxation. The following practice of inner silence is in fact a departure from relaxation and a first step towards actual meditation.

The beginner should never overdo this process since this meditation is quite different from relaxation. With this practice you complete the preliminaries of relaxation and enter into the first phase of meditation. It is only after perfecting this class of dhyana that you should take to further meditations which are higher and deeper in comparison to this one.

Stage 3: Chidakasha awareness

Close the eyes first.
Become aware of chidakasha, the inner space you see behind your forehead.
Go on seeing everything in it.
You will experience various shades of light, stars, illumination and astral figures.
You should remain a witness to these experiences.
The chidakasha or the astral place is before you.
You can project your subconscious mind on it if you have a deep sense of meditation.
Set aside every thought that comes to you.
Remain aware of incoming thoughts.
You are engaged in setting them aside.
At the same time you are aware of what is happening in the astral realms.
If you can do this you can move on to meditation.
Then visions of astral events will follow.
You are standing at the gate.
You are seeing your thoughts come to you.

Your inner chamber is open from all sides for thoughts to enter from any side.
You have to take a central position and from there you have to look everywhere.
From which side is the thought coming?
When you see a particular thought lurking, stop it.
After some time start meditation on your ishta.
If, however, you have even a little success in this sadhana, you will have no necessity to meditate on the ishta.
The form of the ishta will automatically arise from within.
If you do this faithfully you will attain the *nirvichar* stage.
Have constant awareness of chidakasha.
Also see the astral patterns forming over it.
If you observe them for some time, you will understand what we mean by astral patterns.
You will experience various invisible vibrations floating across the chidakasha.
Gradually, you should try to become more and more aware of chidakasha.
Let your consciousness become deep and intense, so much so that you do not feel like taking your mind away from chidakasha even for a moment.
There should be no analysis whatever of experiences on the astral plane.
And thus, when you keep on observing the state of nothingness, you will realize various astral realities which remained out of sight so far. There does come a state of mind when the vast fields of astral realization are left open to you and a whole stock of latent knowledge is apprehended.
When astral figures start floating in chidakasha, at once turn towards the ishta devata and meditate calmly and in silence.
You can repeat the entire process.

Chidakasha Vidya

A POWERFUL TECHNIQUE IN MEDITATION

Of the several techniques of meditation in yoga practice, chidakasha vidya is a powerful and self-absorbing technique. We find reference to chidakasha vidya in the Vedas. In ancient scriptures the truth was indicated broadly but the technique to achieve and arrive at it was always left to be taught by the tradition of master and disciple.

First introduction

Chidakasha vidya is a secret technique of meditation for self-realization. *Vidya* here means dhyana or meditation, and *chidakasha* is the unconscious existence of the mind plus the self. When you close your eyes you see a vast panorama of darkness inside. St. John of the Cross refers to it as 'the dark night of the soul'. This abstract, unperceivable existence of the inner self, finding expression and manifestation in the form of lone and abiding awareness of darkness, is chidakasha in guise.

Darkness (ignorance) covers the light of the soul. The disciple has to penetrate and pass through this darkness until he sees the 'light eternal'. The words of the master will only serve as a guide and the disciple has to travel through the darkness with faith and love in the master's words.

When you sit for the practice of chidakasha vidya, with eyes closed and in a comfortable posture, you will first enter into darkness. Therefore, the Upanishad says, "Those who worship in ignorance enter darkness (sleep) and those who worship meditation also enter the darkness that permeates within when the eyes are closed". But this is not perennial darkness. It is evanescent. It changes.

Symbol manifestation

If you practise chidakasha vidya you will gradually see fog, smoke, darkness, sun, stars, air, fire, fireflies, flying birds, electric sparks, crystal, the moon and many other things. You may see many things according to the impressions hidden deep within you, things that are lying accumulated in the subconscious and unconscious personality. Therefore, an aspirant is generally able to see in the background of chidakasha the above mentioned symbols, either on suggestion from his guide or by his own effort. When the suggestion works the symbols are seen in imagination, but a stage is reached through deep concentration when all these things are actually visualized by the practitioner during meditation. All these symbols are concentrated forms of ideas in the lower mind, and this lower mind reveals itself in a variety of ways.

As you earnestly practise, with faith and devotion, you will see chidakasha illumined and on some glorious day you may receive the 'light of your soul' like a shining lamp. The state is one of enduring bliss and contentment, of unimaginable delight, peace and power.

For the practice of chidakasha vidya you are required to do two things at the very outset. Firstly, you must have unwavering devotion and faith in your guide and master. This is the essential, yet very difficult condition. Secondly, mastery of one meditation posture is also necessary. Chidakasha vidya, apart from its spiritual value, is psychotherapy. It is also the key to God realization. Its psychological aspect would be more attractive, interesting and inspiring to modern readers than the mystical aspect which always unwantedly asserts itself as good and reminds you of God, even if you do not feel the necessity to see God in this life.

Even though your conviction is partially true the good results occuring out of the practice of chidakasha vidya, after a little sacrifice, are worth aspiring for and possessing.

You may well ask if you can change your posture during the meditation? Yes, you may, there is no bar to it, but that will immediately bring your ingoing, upward consciousness down to the physical plane, and it will require a fresh effort to 'go in' again. Besides, the feeling of pain in the limbs, reminding us to change posture, is a hindrance to the inward journey of the consciousness. You cannot remain in the same posture for a long time if you have not perfected asanas. Coming out, even for a few seconds, will mean a fresh start. It is, therefore, advisable that a beginner should aim at perfecting the asanas first.

The best asanas for meditation in order of preference are: siddhasana, siddha yoni asana, padmasana, swastikasana and sukhasana. You should select one of these for yourself and practise it frequently, so that you may get used to it and overcome the pain likely to be caused during meditation practice.

The elasticity and flexibility of the bones and spinal column are to a great extent responsible in securing perfection in asana. Rigidity and stiffness of the bones, limbs and ligaments are neither good for muscular health nor for meditation. These defects will automatically be removed by regular practice of asana and pranayama.

Time for practice

The best time for practice of chidakasha vidya is in the early hours of the morning and at night after taking a bath.

Importance of bathing

A bath with water has much significance and a direct impact on the mind. After bathing the mind feels refreshed. Even a long sleep does not refresh the mind as much as a bath. Neither sleep nor food can give you that emotional and nervous strength and the feeling of being refreshed that a bath gives within a few minutes. Tiredness of body and mind are completely wiped out and the mental state thus acquired is conducive to meditation.

Mystic symbol

What is chidakasha? This term has to be comprehended in its correct manner. The proper significance has to be grasped before you can successfully undertake the practice. *Chidakasha* is made up of two words, *chit* and *akasha*. *Chit* means consciousness, awareness and *akasha* means space. Our awareness extends in time and space and it is a portion of our subjective understanding. Chidakasha very much represents the inner firmament, the awareness which moves in inner space, that is, the consciousness which is all comprehensive.

Western psychologists have tried to probe the human mind and have discovered three layers: the conscious, the subconscious and the unconscious. Indian philosophers speak of the gross, subtle and causal bodies where consciousness remains, and also of the three states of waking, dreaming and sleeping. The fourth state they call transcendental. But these are broad classifications. The ancient sages had realized from experience that there are fourteen planes in which the awareness, that is chit, functions. Your consciousness is on the sensual planes and, therefore, is extrovert. In sleep your consciousness is there, but you are aware of it only when you wake up. This is also the case when you dream. As the chit or the awareness becomes more subtle, it goes to more and more subtle regions till it becomes pure consciousness. Chidakasha vidya is a practice to make the consciousness pure in its entirety. Therefore, when you withdraw your consciousness from the field of gross, outward perception you begin to see symbols and visions. These are the processes within by which the impressions gathered and deposited in the inner recesses of your being (in the causal body or unconscious), slowly come out. Even these experiences, though astral, have an element of grossness about them. You will thus see that chit is awareness, and that the extension of awareness, from a limited range of experience to a wider, purer and more subtle range, is the aim of chidakasha vidya.

There is infinite space within ourselves. When you close your eyes you are able to measure to some extent your infinite existence in the world in the form of consciousness. With eyes closed your vision penetrates deeper. The senses become more refined. Chidakasha is thus the personification of mysticism. With its powers of imagination, thought, speculation and will, it can penetrate into any area of the world. When you dwell within, it is on the plane of chidakasha that you are aware of your existence although you are not able to see your gross material body. This subtle but lively experience of the self and its workings takes place in the background of chidakasha. The infinite, unidimensional, eternal space of chidakasha is a platform for the manifestation of your consciousness.

Yoga anatomy

It is desirable to have an idea of yoga anatomy before trying to understand what chit is. According to yogic anatomy it is said that man's being consists of twenty different elements: five *karmendriyas* (working organs), five *jnanendriyas* (sense organs), five pranas, the four constituents of the *antah karana* and the consciousness or spirit. The antah karana is a collective name for mind, intellect, *chitta* (memory) and the awareness of 'I'. Thus we find that our ancient rishis were fully aware of the unconscious and the subconscious dimensions of man.

Seat of chidakasha

The chit is unidimensional consciousness or awareness of our inner personality. It is a vast treasure house of knowledge of all kinds. It has an all-pervasive record of the past, present and future. Chit is the unending firmament of inward awareness enveloping both the conscious and unconscious existence of man. The seat of chit may roughly be located above the eyebrows in the forehead. There is one consciousness which works through the sense organs while extrovert, and the same is turned inwards when we close the doors of our outer sense organs through physical and mental efforts. The chit appears to function through the apparatus of the mind and the intellect but it is beyond their reach. You can experience it only when mind and intellect both cease their normal functioning in connection with the senses. To have a thorough understanding of the chit is essential, since it is the root cause of all human activities. To locate the chidakasha, you must hold your consciousness somewhere in the cavity of the skull just behind the bones of the forehead. Have an unwavering grip over the point where your consciousness gathers while closing the eyes. Very often this seat is imagined in the hollow of the forehead's bony cavity. Therefore, while concentrating on chidakasha, the space behind the forehead should serve as a material footing on which to centre your consciousness.

Practice of chidakasha dharana

The practice of chidakasha dharana is divided into five stages as follows:

Stage 1

The first stage consists of your watching the darkness that envelops the chidakasha when you close your eyes. You have to continue to watch it carefully as a witness, seeing some drama unfolding before your mind's eye until the second stage is reached.

Stage 2

In the second stage you will see the darkness interspersed by a variety of colours – red, yellow, blue and so on.

It may happen that the darkness is replaced by a colour like the golden dawn.

Your attention must be centred on watching this interplay

of colours, neither trying to think, nor understand or analyze them. Continue doing so for some time. Then go further.

Stage 3

In the third stage, let the consciousness penetrate deeply through the veil of darkness or the play of colours.
Make it deeper.
Your concentration is getting more intense.
Here is the basis of mental telepathy.
Therefore, you have to be careful.
Intensify your concentration, and at the same witness the flight of consciousness in the 'dark night of the soul'.
As the practice intensifies you will come across rare experiences.
Continue this for some time.

Stage 4

The fourth stage consists of having an overall survey of chidakasha.
Above, below, at the front, back and sides, consciousness becomes all-pervasive.
It behaves as if it is a person in search of something, gazing all around himself and fully alert to what he is doing.
So you must survey chidakasha for some time, at the same time carefully retaining the awareness that you are doing so.
Then come to the fifth stage.

Stage 5

The fifth stage consists of putting yourself in the centre of chidakasha.
Visualize the inner firmament or chidakasha and then try to be in the centre of it.
Your awareness will then become more subtle and penetrating by practice.

After this, meditate on your ishta devata in chidakasha for a short time and then end the practice.

Conclusion

Through the practice of chidakasha dharana, you can experience the existence of chit very well. For therapeutic value and the prevention of physical and mental diseases, you have to reach to this depth of your personality. You have to approach the chit for fulfilment of your desire.

It is very difficult for anyone to explain this science of subtle experiences and experiments in words. We have tried to give theoretical details as far as possible but your knowledge will be complete only when you sit daily for meditation and, after some months of practice, begin to comprehend it as well as to start experiencing the presence of this abstract astral matter.

The Psychic Horizon

ITS EXPLORATION

Occultists, spiritualists, saints, sages, adepts and the scriptures bear testimony to the existence of several other universes which are apart from ours. Supernatural experience in the daily life of thousands of individuals further assures us that there are mysterious planes beyond the perception of our physical eyes.

Besides these, we see almost daily many passing to the other world through the gateway of death. Do we still need more proof? If so, then better sit in quietude. Think for a moment that you are going to die in the next moment. Don't be afraid. Closely watch your thoughts. What will happen if you die? How will you feel? You, who are just now alive, full of consciousness, full of bright intellect and wisdom, will you extinguish into nothingness? No! Never will you feel that you will not outlive the death of the body. Your consciousness will remain somewhere else and that is in the psychic world, the unseen, the invisible world.

This is why we firmly believe that we have not this world alone to live in. There are other worlds also where we live and move in our subtle body, which is comprized of finer elements. This visible world of ours is made up of five gross elements named *prithvi* (earth), *apas* (water), *agni* (fire), *vayu* (air) and *akasha* (ether).

The psychic, astral planes are made up of ethereal elements having very fine vibrations which cannot be grasped or caught in any way by our present senses, which are used in comprehending the coarser vibrations in comparison to those of the *sukshma lokas* (subtle planes).

The power of the human intellect and energy is just like a lighted candle that removes the darkness. If you put this energy to the study and practice of fine arts you will be known as an artist. If you direct it towards music you will be known as a musician. If you put it towards scientific research you will be known as a scientist. The same energy, when employed for the exploration of the unseen powers and laws of nature, is known as yoga. Yoga is a school of thought which teaches the technique by which to transcend the limitations of the body and the mind. One who employs or utilizes his energy for the study and practice of yoga, broadens and improves his vision by redirecting the downward trend of his energy.

When we check the energy leaking through the sensuous enjoyments of worldly things which have no permanent value, we feel stronger, more energetic and more powerful. When one meditates on some object, or tries to know the hidden truth behind the apparent, he uses this accumulated strength to achieve success. His vision and power of perception become so keen that he can look through the thick covering of matter.

The psychic world we talk of is very near, yet very far, in the sense that it is inaccessible to the common mass of people. Yet one who is willing to toil and tire will be given, or finds the access. The knowledge acquired therefrom is to be utilized for the upliftment of mankind and not for personal benefit.

Perseverance and personal effort are the prerequisites for practice. But when a man acquires supernatural faculties he should not entertain the desires which worldly people possess. He has to dwell in a state of super-consciousness; at least he should attempt to do so while trying to get the passport. He must not brood over food, fashion, fame, politics, power or money.

There is no harm in this, but the utmost energy is to be preserved and utilized for yoga practices. The aspirant or student willing to explore the land of the invisible must remain single-minded all the while, and should carefully keep himself away from adverse influences which may undo the result so far achieved.

It is easy to obtain the gate pass to the ethereal regions provided you detach your mind from mundane interest. Unless you cut the strings of attachment for worldly objects you cannot attach yourself to the objects of the supernatural world. This is why the scriptures and saints advocate *vairagya* (detachment). This can be achieved if we cut short the emotions and thoughts constantly flowing towards all types of nonsense, from silicon chips to jet planes and space ships. If we do so, we can gradually develop the faculty of hearing the voice of silence, seeing the vision of the unseen, and smelling the inodorous.

The secret is this: there is a vast panorama of life, a vast universe, an enormous divine store of knowledge of everything, even beyond this earth. We are living in that world, yet we are not aware. We are perhaps not conscious of those things because our whole energy is diverted in acquiring ephemeral things of this world alone. We live for bread, education, power, television, bangles and many other things. Who cares to labour for the knowledge of the supernatural or the divine? But those who care, even a little, to have the knowledge of these supernatural things, gain valuable benefits. These people are known in the history of mankind as saints, seers, yogis and adepts. The adepts have been careful to arrange the handing down of their art and skill to successors. This is why this knowledge has been preserved despite several seeming contradictions.

If you want to know something about the psychic land, first be prepared to take up and regularly pursue some practice. Get up at 2 a.m. Practise this technique which is preliminary preparation for the beginner at the outset, but which will ultimately lead you towards the psychic land.

Technique for exploration

Preparation: For this purpose you must have one room exclusively for your own use. It is desirable that the atmosphere be kept free from outer influences. Take an old hanging calendar. On the back of the calendar put a black spot with a diameter of three-quarters of an inch. Light a candle. Arrange your seat near the wall either on a chair or on the ground. Hang the calendar on the wall so that, when you are sitting, the black spot will be at eye level. Put a small table on the left of your chair or seat. Burn a candle and put it on the table when you intend to sit for practice.

Practice

Sit for practice at 2 a.m. daily.

Fix your gaze on the black spot. Look with full concentration. Intently gaze, relentlessly gaze.

Go on looking at the black spot. In the beginning, if your eyes water and get tired, rest by closing the eyes for ten seconds. Then again start gazing at the spot.

While attempting to gaze at the spot you must see the spot alone and nothing else.

White light will surround the spot as soon as you start gazing with full concentration.

This light will move and you will be tempted to pursue the white light. You should refrain from doing so.

Stick to gazing at the black spot until your mind becomes blank and you see nothing. Nothing whatsoever.

At this time you will receive many thought currents which will distract you from your mission and pursuit.

You should remain indifferent.

Don't allow the thoughts to enter your mind.

Go on looking at the spot until it vanishes and you start seeing some figure, either with eyes closed or eyes open.

This practice cuts off the link of the mind with the surrounding world and at once places it at the disposal of the subconscious powers which are directly linked with the psychic land.

Atma Anubhuti Yoga

SELF-AWARENESS

Self-awareness is to be evolved in stages and by this process you will ultimately realize the existence of a power within. During the yogic practices of japa and meditation you can develop it. After proper development self-awareness becomes a reality and an experience.

Before explaining the practice of self-awareness let us state a few important points.

Remember the words: body consciousness, pranic consciousness, mental consciousness, astral consciousness, causal consciousness and disembodied consciousness. You should remember all these six phases of consciousness.

When you sit in a posture the first consciousness is called body consciousness. Then you slowly breathe in and out. After some time you will feel that bodily consciousness is diminishing and you are becoming more conscious of the ingoing and outgoing breath. You gradually become all the more aware of the flow of prana. As a result of this, after some time, pranic consciousness becomes predominant and body consciousness is extinct. At that stage you will feel that you are just breathing, breathing and breathing.

When you are aware of breath consciousness, that is, pranic consciousness, and when it becomes predominant, then it is called 'bodily unconsciousness'. You become unconscious of your body. You are conscious only of the flow of prana.

Now to that pranic consciousness add the mantra *om* or *soham* and become conscious of the mantra. Then you feel *so* with the ingoing breath and *ham* with outgoing breath. After some time you will become unaware of the two streams of breath; simple *soham* will remain in your awareness. When this becomes intense you will have visions.

As you see visions, mental consciousness begins to fuse into astral awareness. At this stage all forms of ajapa will be consumed by an ever-growing astral consciousness. You will land in a plane which is beyond the mental plane.

Here the suspension of individual consciousness will take place, as a result of which the aspirant will enter into deep slumber and become unaware even of the process. Those who practise this in shavasana will revive awareness only in the morning, but those practising in padmasana may experience this awareness any time.

Every spiritual practitioner can experience and attain the state of astral consciousness by simple guidance and correct practice. But when the self goes to the unconscious, the aspirant will have different experiences. He will then experience cyclic movements: slumber, visions, dreams, again slumber, and so on. Here he moves between the astral and causal spheres of the self. Beyond this no one can go alone. This is the phase of complete darkness, where you are not aware of anything like time or space. There is absolute suspension of every activity of the mind. There is no functioning of the will. As a result, the aspirant returns to the realm of visions, then suddenly, or gradually, back to mental, pranic and body consciousness. In yogic language, we call it coming and going or taking birth again and again, which really means revival of consciousness.

If you want to go beyond this phase of consciousness instruction alone is not sufficient. Guides, books or satsang will not help you. Here a guru is essential, one who can create light from darkness. The guru is the dispeller of the darkness which is pervading chidakasha. He is the one who takes you through the chamber of unconsciousness, which in yoga is the 'fifth chamber', and through which no aspirant can pierce without guru's grace. For no sooner does he enter it, than he becomes totally unconscious of himself. There is no trace in him of willpower. Therefore, in the fifth chamber he needs someone to carry him through. When the aspirant sleeps in the fifth chamber of meditation, he does not hear with the ears but follows the guru's instructions. His guru's commands are received through ajna chakra, and none except those whose ajna chakra has begun developing can listen to the guru's commands. Here is the general method:

1. Meditate on the body and transcend the body.
2. Meditate on the prana and transcend the prana.
3. Meditate on the mind and transcend the mind.
4. Meditate on the visions and transcend them.

After this is done, those who wish to do away with the guru should meditate on the unconscious self and transcend that also. However, this method is not so simple. It is easier to contact a guru, although he is a rare commodity, than it is to transcend this chamber merely by concentration and mindfulness alone.

Practice

Stretch your legs and relax, but with full consciousness.
You should be aware of your entire body.
Just be sure that you are mindful of the body.
Just entertain the simple thought, 'I am aware of my body'. Your mind should think only of that in unbroken awareness. There should be a continuous awareness of the body.
If you hear any sound, like that of a radio or a car, be indifferent. Do not sit for meditation with a vow that you will not be disturbed.
If you create such a mental attitude, external factors will disturb you very much.
Once you step into the field of mental consciousness nothing can disturb you.

When you practise body awareness you can experience the first stage of sleep. But hold on to your consciousness along the borderline between the body and the mind.

When you meditate you will distinctly see the demarcation line. You can hold your consciousness on the borderline.

If you meditate on the body and hold on to the borderline, you will experience the phases of pranic, mental and astral consciousness.

Then you will go on to the unconscious state.

If you cannot, somehow, hold on to the body consciousness, you will surely go into unconsciousness, but there will be no vision. Therefore, continue your awareness without a break. Constant unbroken consciousness.

You can practise this with eyes open or closed, but it is better with closed eyes.

Further details

If you practise in any posture, you will have to visualize the body. Please do not go into details. Do not say, 'I am erect, I am fat,' etc. Simply, 'I am'. While you practise, if you feel drowsy, awaken a great deal of willpower in yourself and say mentally, 'I am'. In that stage only body consciousness will diminish. You will not be totally unconscious of the body, but the self-consciousness of the body will diminish. This is bodiless consciousness. There is consciousness of 'I am' but there is no body consciousness at all.

When you sleep you feel that sleep is coming to you, but you do not think of the body although you have the body then. This is nearly the same experience. Please understand this very well. Otherwise you will have two difficulties. You will either revive body consciousness or you will sleep. You have to be careful. It is as if you are walking on a tight-rope.

This 'I am' changes into 'I am Brahman' – God. First you become aware of yourself. When you become steady in this practice, you become aware of supreme consciousness. This is realization, not mere intellectual conception. In the sixth chamber this embodied consciousness is to be transcended.

The Link of Consciousness

THE TECHNIQUE FOR ITS DISCOVERY

That which is in me is in all. That which I am is in everybody else. This is the knowledge to be acquired and experienced in life. The essence of all creation is the same. It should be my abiding experience that the entire creation is inseparably linked with *me*. For I must know and realize that far beyond the mind, the body and the senses, there is an unseen link which holds in itself the different beads of the visible and invisible creation. We talk of 'blood relations', 'community relations', 'social relations' and relations of different kinds. Let us add to those different kinds of relations, a relation of a distinct and singular type, which is abiding and universal – *the relation of the inner self* – which implies that all are, in essence, tied by the unity of one self.

A realization of this knowledge sustains our thoughts and gives shape to our behaviour towards fellow-beings in all walks of life: with relatives, friends, so-called enemies and the global village. Let us at least try to feel for a while when we are amidst them, that *that* which is in me is in them too, and that in essence we are one and the same. There is an unbroken unity in seemingly divided variety.

What is the method to realize this knowledge and practise it in this life? Let us experiment in this way. Take the case of your father, brother, sister, husband, wife or friend, who appears to be standing aloof and away from you in thought, principle and faith. Set in rotation this knowledge (which you have taken pains to acquire), that *that* which is in you is in him or her too, that the essence of both of you is ever and for all times the same. Let this knowledge rotate within you first until it has reached higher frequencies, or until you actually feel within you, that *that* which is in you is in him or her too.

When this knowledge gains higher frequency and intensity by the practice of *right meditation on the unity of essence* an unseen link will soon be established. You will feel as if it were running through both of you. As a result, the other person would somehow become awakened to your thought, principle, faith, overcoming these separative factors. The points of difference will vanish and common points will emerge. The person will begin to commune with you in an enlightened manner. This phenomenon is known as *spiritual union*, as opposed to physical or mental difference.

Let us take the case of any animal which appears to be standing away and aloof from the centre of your abilities, knowledge and reach, because of its immature and undeveloped psycho-physiological constitution. Here too, set this knowledge in rotation that *that* which is in you is there too, that the inner essence of both of you is ever the same. Let this knowledge rotate within you in the form of right meditation until you actually see, feel and experience the existence of the inner link running in and through both of you. When this link has been seen by means of the right meditation on the unity of essence, an unseen communion will be effected within both the selves.

That which is in me is in all, that is the real knowledge which we propose to impress on your mind. We would have you realize the undying link of the soul, the substratum of all beings. Also realize that you can work on them to move in accordance with your faith, principle and behaviour.

However, keep this resolve before you always: that you are not going to make use of this knowledge for selfish ends or unholy intentions, or to possess personalities. Forever hold before your mind's eye that you are making this experiment in order to realize the essential and underlying soul or *Ishwara* who is, as it were, interwoven into everything in this universe. You should forever remain awake to the pure and elevating principle that you are conducting this experiment on others so that you may realize that *that* which is in you is in all; that beyond the body, thoughts, emotions, sensations and unconsciousness which are diverse in each being, there exists one *common unseen* principle running through and permeating everything in this vast universe.

But let this be done through the medium of meditation alone, without any personal contact through the body or mind. Pure meditation, devoid of impure motives but activated by chaste desire, will certainly lead to success. If this experiment is not conducted with a pure mind, in a spirit of an ennobled ideal, then there is a danger of the subject becoming obsessed and reacting in a harmful fashion, quite contrary to your expectation. Therefore, try not to convert an enemy into a friend and in all experiments concentrate on the discovery of the missing link of consciousness. One who has discovered this is a yogi, because he has joined and cemented these different factors by the realization of *oneness*.

Men who harbour hatred, or who are actuated by malice or similar notions, should keep away from this practice. They should first eradicate their wrong emotions by love, charity, understanding, sympathy, compassion and friendliness. Men of passion must also refrain till they have overcome passion through various other yogic practices and celibacy. Men of greed must also avoid this practice till they have overcome their greed by contentment and *tyaga* (sacrifice).

That which is in me is in all: this knowledge should take us nearer to the field of unity. It makes us one with all and develops divine virtues within ourselves. Finally it helps us realize our goal of God realization or the experience of cosmic consciousness.

Bihar Yoga

AN OVERVIEW OF ITS DEVELOPMENT

This chapter has been included to give the reader an overview of the history, evolution and current implementation of Bihar Yoga, both within India and abroad.

Origins of Bihar Yoga

The Bihar Yoga (or Satyananda Yoga) tradition is the system of yoga developed and expounded by Swami Satyananda Saraswati and his successor Swami Niranjanananda Saraswati, based on texts and teachings of the traditions of Samkhya, Vedanta, Yoga and Tantra handed down through the lineage of ancient sannyasa.

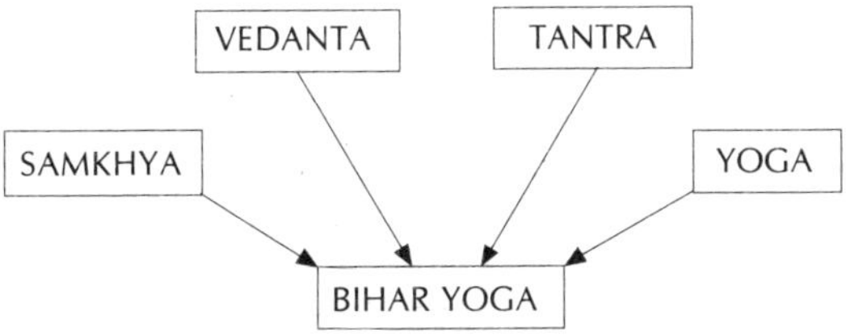

Swami Satyananda sought to revive the ancient yogic sciences and offer them in a renewed form to suit the needs of modern times. Thus Bihar Yoga emerged and evolved from a rich spiritual heritage. These ancient traditions and texts of yoga continue to be explored and precious knowledge extracted, aiming towards the total development of human nature and personality in the field of yoga. The techniques of Bihar Yoga integrate the wisdom of the past with today's needs.

The integral approach of Bihar Yoga

Bihar Yoga adopts the attitudes of *jnana yoga* (the path of knowledge), *bhakti yoga* (the path of channelling the emotions in a positive direction), *karma yoga* (the path of selfless service) and other yogas (including *hatha yoga, raja yoga, mantra yoga, kundalini yoga* and *kriya yoga*) which enable practitioners to frame the different aspects of their lives in a way which is conducive to spiritual growth.

- *Jnana yoga* is the process of converting intellectual knowledge into practical wisdom. It is the discovery of human dharma in relation to nature, human society and the universe. Jnana yoga is described by the tradition as a means to obtain the highest meditative state and inner knowledge, through training the awareness as a discipline.
- *Bhakti yoga* is the path of channelling the emotions and feelings to realize the transcendental and divine nature inherent in every human being. It brings about the transformation of emotions into a positive expression. Many people describe this as the yoga of devotion and give it a religious bent; however, it is through bhakti yoga that it becomes possible to experience the unity of all life.
- *Karma yoga* is a system which develops immunity to the reactive and negative components of an action. This awareness of action leads to a greater ability to manage mental expressions and manifestations in the form of desires, ambitions, ego and other components of the personality. Karma yoga is a sadhana and not a philosophy. It implies living and acting in the present, having gained experience from the past, without worry or concern for the future. The state of karma yoga can be attained through *seva* (selfless involvement in all activities), the spirit of which can be imbibed under the guidance of a competent master.

The approach of Bihar Yoga integrates the whole person, not just the physical body or intellect. Emphasis is placed on awareness and practitioners are encouraged to explore and learn about the various aspects of their personality through yogic practices. Positive transformation is a natural process which occurs as a result of regular practice performed with full awareness, not through forcing the mind and body to the limit and beyond.

Inspirers of Bihar Yoga

The roots of the Bihar Yoga tradition lie in Rishikesh, in the foothills of the Himalayas, where the renowned yogic master, Swami Sivananda taught an integral approach to yoga. From his original inspiration to its present day application around the world, Bihar Yoga has evolved into an integrated system of yoga able to address today's needs within the community. Through the teachings and guidance of successive yogic masters and inspirers, the ancient yogic wisdom continues to filter through to all who seek yoga in their lives.

Swami Sivananda Saraswati wrote hundreds of books and articles on yoga and spirituality throughout his life, which continue to introduce and instil yogic values in the minds and hearts of the public. His emphasis was on breaking down the barriers that separated the needy from the yogic teachings that could help them, whether this took the form of yoga for health, peace of mind or spiritual aspiration.

Swami Sivananda's concept of yoga is summed up in his *ashtanga* (eightfold) yoga system: serve, love, give, purify, do good, be good, meditate, realize. This ideology continues to guide the work of Bihar Yoga.

Swami Satyananda Saraswati spread Swami Sivananda's message of yoga to the world through his disciples as well as his authoritative teachings and writings. After the completion of twelve years training in Rishikesh he spent nine years traversing India, observing human suffering at all strata of society. Thus he concluded that yoga could provide the solution for the problems and needs of modern man.

Through the establishment of Bihar School of Yoga and other yogic institutions (see Bihar Yoga Family), Swami Satyananda was able to provide centres for teaching the principles and practices of yoga and spiritual life. His sannyasins became the pioneers of research into yoga, exploring such areas as the benefits of yoga in relation to health, the mind and human evolution.

Although Swami Satyanada has now withdrawn from the active role of a yogic guru, and lives in semi-seclusion as a paramahamsa sannyasin, his inspiration continues to guide the application and development of Bihar Yoga.

Swami Niranjanananda Saraswati continues the work of his guru and paramguru, addressing the changing needs of the community and incorporating yoga into these areas (see Social Development). He guides and inspires the many yoga centres initiated by Swami Satyananda in India and around the world, through extensive travels, conventions and programs. New centres of yogic teaching and activities are also developed in those countries or areas where there is a growing interest in yoga.

In 1994 Swami Niranjan founded Bihar Yoga Bharati, the world's first gurukul[1] university of yoga, with the aim of preserving and regenerating the yogic sciences by combining academic and scientific methodology with a spiritual vision. With his creation of Bal Yoga Mitra Mandal (Children's Yoga Fellowship) in 1995, yoga was introduced to children (see Bihar Yoga Family).

Development of Bihar Yoga practices

The teaching and training of yoga developed by Bihar Yoga introduce the following points:

- It promotes physical and mental balance and well-being through classical hatha yoga and raja yoga techniques.

---

[1] Whereas a university focuses solely on academic goals, the gurukul university combines both intellectual and experiential learning, aiming towards the holistic growth of the student, with emphasis on mental and spiritual development.

- It provides mental and emotional stability through the progressive develoment of pratyahara, dharana, dhyana, mantra yoga, karma yoga, raja yoga and bhakti yoga.
- Self-discovery and inner awakening are enabled through classical kriyas and kundalini yoga.
- It culminates in prosperity[2] and harmony at all levels through wisdom (jnana yoga).

Scientific experimentation and research are central themes of Bihar Yoga. From the very beginning Swami Satyananda experimented with knowledge from the scriptures, extracted what was relevant and reintroduced it in a practical form. Asanas were systematized and grouped according to position and sequence. One important contribution was the pawanmuktasana part 1 (anti-rheumatic), part 2 (anti-gastric) and part 3 (shakti bandha or energy- releasing) series. The introduction of the shatkarmas (purification practices) was another important contribution of Bihar Yoga.

In the past the practices of pranayama had been taught only to a select few as part of higher yogic practice, but Swami Satyananda reintroduced pranayama as part of daily yoga sadhana. The sequence in which pranayama is taught today by many yoga schools was developed by the Bihar Yoga tradition.

The physiological and psychological effects of mudras and bandhas were examined and systematized. Swami Satyananda was the first to explain the role of mudras and bandhas scientifically. In Bihar Yoga, mudras and bandhas have been combined with many asana, pranayama and meditation techniques, thus enhancing the pranic effects.

The practice of yoga nidra, devised by Swami Satyananda in early 1964 from traditional tantric practices, has had a major impact on the world of yoga. Yoga nidra systematically induces complete physical, mental and emotional relaxation, and can be used by beginners, intermediate and advanced practitioners. It is widely acknowledged as an

---

[2] Here 'prosperity' means the wealth of contentment, the prosperity of spirit.

important therapeutic technique for stress-induced disorders, as well as for the transformation of personality and, ultimately, for spiritual evolution.

Many concentration and meditation techniques have been developed by Bihar Yoga from the ancient scriptures. Swami Satyananda developed various meditations from the tantras which he taught in the form of antar mouna, ajapa japa, trataka, chidakasha dharana and prana vidya. The practices of pratyahara (sense withdrawal), dharana (one-pointedness) and dhyana (meditative awareness) derived from the Upanishads, the tantras and other traditions, have been classified, taught and published. All the techniques have different levels and stages of practice as classified by the Bihar Yoga tradition.

The techniques of kriya yoga were propagated by Swami Satyananda from secret teachings described in the yoga and tantra shastras. He distilled the essence of the practices, giving them a definite form and sequence of practice. The kriya yoga system, as taught by Bihar Yoga, is one of two systems of kriya yoga recognized the world over, the other being that of Paramahamsa Yogananda.

In Bihar Yoga emphasis is laid upon developing the faculty of awareness to gain maximum benefit from practices and to accelerate one's conscious evolution. For example, during asana practice, aspirants gradually expand their awareness from the gross to the more subtle dimensions. Physical awareness is followed by breath awareness, mental awareness and ultimately pranic awareness, as the gradual expansion of awareness occurs.

The development of the ability to 'witness', which further expands the faculty of awareness, is another important aspect of Bihar Yoga. The ability to stand back from all that one is experiencing, whether physically, mentally, emotionally or psychically, is the basis of successful yogic sadhana, whatever activity one may be engaged in. Witnessing also develops the personal discipline of acting rather than reacting during the course of life's varying situations.

A third important aspect of Bihar Yoga is the emphasis on adopting a yogic lifestyle, which develops optimism and creativity within the individual character.

YOGIC SOCIAL SUPPORT

Bihar School of Yoga has succeeded in bringing yoga into the lives of professionals, intellectuals and academics, and also into the infrastructure of industries, private and public undertakings, companies, medical and other social institutions. From this viewpoint, Bihar School of Yoga and other yoga centres around the world have been organizing yoga programs to promote inner harmony, work proficiency and self-discipline within society. The following programs are a part of the school's social and human resource development scheme:

- Stress management and business management programs.
- Yoga health management training and research.
- Special yoga training programs for the military, prisons, police, railways, private and public organizations, sporting associations, educational institutes, medical colleges and hospitals.
- Camps, seminars, conferences, symposiums, workshops, forums and gatherings on yoga throughout India and the world.
- Rural upliftment.

In India today, yoga programs incorporating Bihar Yoga are currently being applied within private and public sector industries, such as the Indian Oil Corporation, Coal India Ltd., National Thermal Power Corporation, Oil & Natural Gas Corporation, the Steel Authority of India, Hindustan Paper Corporation, Hindustan Copper Ltd., and many others.

Internationally, the application of Bihar Yoga addresses a range of current problems within society, for example: addiction, drug and alcohol rehabilitation, the physically and mentally disabled (including children), troubled or homeless teenagers, the elderly, prisoners, abused women, HIV-positive patients, autistic adults and creative development through yoga nidra. These special community programs are run in addition to regular, ongoing yoga classes and programs.

Yoga in educational institutions

Special training programs have been provided in government schools for students and teachers to promote sound health, a positive, optimistic and creative attitude and increased receptivity, and learning and memory proficiency. These courses have been conducted in the states of Bihar, Orissa, Uttar Pradesh and Madhya Pradesh. At the request of the government of Bihar, from 1985–1987, 2,000 secondary school teachers were trained in the Bihar Yoga system for the purpose of educating students in yoga techniques.

Yoga training in medical colleges

At the request of the Ministry of Health, government of Bihar, medically qualified sannyasins and yoga teachers have conducted training courses in yoga therapy for medical students and doctors at the medical colleges of Bhagalpur, Patna, Nalanda, Dharbanga, Ranchi and Dhanbad, and at medical institutions in other states on demand.

Yoga training for military and police

Specialized yoga training camps are being conducted for instructors from the army to improve physical, mental and emotional fitness, and to increase the endurance of the combat troops at Danapur, Bikaner, Jabalpur, Mhow, and at Siachen Glacier in the Himalayan region. Bihar School of Yoga also trains instructors from sixteen units of the Bihar Military Police.

Yoga camps and programs

Sannyasins and yoga teachers hold regular camps and programs nationally. A typical yoga camp has two practical class sessions, one from 6.30 to 8.00 a.m., and another from 3.00 to 4.00 p.m. The morning session consists of asana and pranayama and the afternoon session consists of meditation (pratyahara) and mantra yoga. There may be lectures, satsangs, kirtans and workshops during the day and evening on relevant themes.

Yoga in sport

At the request of the Sports Authority of India (SAI), short and longer term courses have been conducted for sportspersons, coaches and physical training teachers to improve physical and mental proficiency.

Yoga in rural development

Trained sannyasins, yoga teachers and volunteers go to remote villages and rural areas throughout the state of Bihar to introduce the Bihar Yoga system for the welfare and improvement of tribal and indigenous people. These courses focus on rural health, lifestyle, character and habits.

BIHAR YOGA FAMILY

International Yoga Fellowship Movement (IYFM)

This institution was conceived by Swami Satyananda during his travels in India as a *parivrajaka* (wandering) sannyasin. His inspiration was to establish a global yoga family comprised of people dedicated to the lifestyle and spirit of yoga. To enable this, he founded the International Yoga Fellowship Movement in 1956. From humble beginnings, the movement spread to carry the message of yoga from door to door and from shore to shore. Its mandate was to help people from every section of society, not only in a spiritual and yogic way, but also physically and socially.

The International Yoga Fellowship Movement began as a philosophical movement and later, as people became more interested in the lifestyle, philosophy and practice it taught, the Bihar School of Yoga was established as its head office.

This became the focal point for people wanting to learn the principles and practices of yoga and spiritual life. Today, with Swami Niranjanananda as Paramacharya, the International Yoga Fellowship Movement has become a global community which unites, inspires and coordinates the family of practitioners who propagate Bihar Yoga (or Satyananda Yoga) all over the world.

Bihar School of Yoga (BSY)

Bihar School of Yoga was founded in 1964 by Swami Satyananda to impart yogic training to householders and sannyasins alike. The yoga techniques developed are a synthesis of many approaches to personal development, based on traditional vedantic, tantric and yogic teachings in conjunction with contemporary physical and mental health sciences.

Today, the Paramacharya of Bihar School of Yoga is Swami Niranjanananda. The yogic techniques are being further developed and taught by Bihar School of Yoga and it also guides yoga research projects and medical investigative research in association with hospitals and other organizations.

Sivananda Math (SM)

This institution is registered as a social and charitable society. It was founded by Swami Satyananda in 1984 in memory of his guru, Swami Sivananda of Rishikesh. Its aim is to facilitate the upliftment of the weaker and underdeveloped sections of society, especially in rural areas. This is undertaken by following the precepts of *seva* (service), *karuna* (compassion), *prem* (love) and *sneha* (affection) espoused by Swami Sivananda.

Each year, during November and December, a special program called Sita Kalyanam is organized by Sivananda Math and held in Rikhia, a rural area in the new state of Jharkhand (formerly part of Bihar). This event provides the opportunity for people from all around the world to participate in and support the activities and projects of Sivananda Math.

Yoga Research Foundation (YRF)

The Yoga Research Foundation is a research institute founded by Swami Satyananda in 1984, with the aim of conducting scientific and medical research to define the role of yogic management in such diseases as: respiratory disorders, cardiac problems, digestive disorders, pregnancy, arthritis, spondylosis, blood pressure, gynaecological problems, diabetes, cancer, HIV-positive and drug addiction, etc.

Today, Swami Niranjanananda is the chief patron of the Foundation. YRF aims to provide an accurate assessment of the practices of different branches of yoga within a scientific framework, and to establish yoga as an essential science for the development of mankind. At present the foundation is working on projects in the areas of fundamental research and clinical research. It is also studying the effects of yoga on proficiency improvement in various social projects, e.g. army, prisoners, children. These projects are being carried out in affiliated centres worldwide.

YRF's future plans include literary, scriptural, medical and scientific investigations into other little-known aspects of yoga for physical health, mental well-being and spiritual upliftment.

Sri Panchdashnam Paramahamsa Alakh Bara (PPAB)

The Sri Panchdashnam Paramahamsa Alakh Bara was established by Swami Niranjanananda in 1991 at Rikhia, Deoghar, Jharkhand. Rikhia is the *tapobhoomi* (sadhana place) of Swami Satyananda. He settled there in 1989 after travelling through the *siddha tirthas* (pilgrimage centres) of India. In Rikhia, Swami Satyananda lived in seclusion and performed higher vedic sadhanas. An infrastructure developed around him which is now recognized as Paramahamsa Alakh Bara. Its aim is to uphold the ideals of sannyasa and sadhana. At the Paramahamsa Alakh Bara sannyasins are guided to follow the path walked by the paramahamsa sannyasins of the past. Training is imparted through direct transmission between guru and disciple. The vision developed is of compassion and love for humanity, maintaining the aim of spiritual life and communing with nature as a part of cosmic creation.

Bihar Yoga Bharati (BYB)

Bihar Yoga Bharati was founded by Swami Niranjanananda in 1994 and recognized as a deemed university in 2000. It is the first university in the world to impart a comprehensive yogic education with provision for MA, MSc, MPhil, PhD, DSc and DLitt. BYB presently offers a four month Certificate Course in Yogic Studies, one year undergraduate and postgraduate Diploma Courses in Yogic Studies, a one year postgraduate Diploma Course in Yoga Ecology, and two year postgraduate courses in Yoga Philosophy, Yoga Psychology and Applied Yogic Science.

BYB admits students with a broad range of interests and backgrounds. Along with yogic education, the spirit of *seva* (selfless service), *samarpan* (dedication) and *karuna* (compassion) is imbibed by the students. BYB is a residential institution where students live in an ashram environment and imbibe yogic lifestlye and training as part of the gurukul (family of the guru).

Internationally, BYB is developing satellite academies in Australia and Greece, which are aiming for full government accreditation in the near future.

Bal Yoga Mitra Mandal (BYMM)

Bal Yoga Mitra Mandal (Children's Yoga Fellowship) is an organization of the children, for the children, run by the children. BYMM was founded by Swami Niranjanananda in 1995 on the initiative of seven school children and a college student. By 2002 BYMM had trained 350 child yoga propagators, 400 child yoga instructors and 1,000 child yoga demonstrators, who had in turn introduced yoga to 56,000 children nationwide.

BYMM is dedicated to:

- Development of the total personality of children between the ages of 7 to 14.
- Training of child yoga propagators, instructors and demonstrators.
- Conducting and coordinating research in the field of yogic education.

BYMM has five major operational groups: yoga learning group, yoga training group, personality development group, research administration group and parent/teacher group.

BYMM has imparted yoga training in 300 schools of India, and since 1997 has conducted the biggest children's yoga festival in the world with over 5,000 children participating every year.

Yoga Publications Trust (YPT)

Yoga Publications Trust (YPT) was established by Swami Niranjanananda in 2000. It is an organization devoted to the dissemination and promotion of yogic and allied knowledge – psychology (ancient and modern), ecology, medicine, vedic, upanishadic, tantric darshanas, philosophies (Eastern and Western), mysticism and spirituality – nationally and internationally through the distribution of books, magazines, audio and video cassettes and multimedia presentations.

YPT is primarily concerned with publishing textbooks in the areas of yoga philosophy, yoga psychology and applied yogic science, research materials, practice texts and the inspiring talks of eminent spiritual personalities and authors aimed at the upliftment of humanity by means of the eternal yogic knowledge, lifestyle and practice.

Glossary

Agni – the gross fire element.

Agnisar dhauti – an exercise in which the abdominal muscles are expanded and contracted while the breath is held outside the body, stimulating proper intestinal peristalsis.

Ahimsa – non-injury in thought and deed.

Ajapa Gayatri – spontaneous repetition of the *soham* mantra.

Ajapa japa – spontaneous repetition of a mantra.

Ajna chakra – the psychic centre at the top of the spinal column in the brain, at the level of the eyebrow centre.

Akasha – the ether element.

Akasha vani – the language of the soul; 'inner voice'.

Anadi vasana – beginningless instincts and desires.

Anahata chakra – psychic centre at the level of the heart region, in the spine.

Anandamaya kosha – the bliss-body; the most subtle of the five sheaths of the human spirit.

Annamaya kosha – the most gross of the five sheaths of the human spirit; the physical or food body.

Antah karana – collective name for the mind (*manas*), intellect (*buddhi*), memory (*smaran*) and the awareness of 'I' (*ahamkara*).

Antar mouna – inner silence.

Antaranga – internal 'limb' or part; refers to the esoteric practices of raja yoga viz. pratyahara, dharana, dhyana and samadhi.

Apana – one of the five manifestations of prana in the human body; associated with the outgoing breath.

Apas – the gross water element.

Ardha Matsyendrasana – the half pose of yogi Matsyendra; the half spinal twist posture.

Asana – yogic posture; any comfortable bodily pose.

Ashtanga yoga – yoga of the eightfold path; raja yoga.

Baddha padmasana – tied lotus pose.

Bahiranga – external 'limb' or part, refers to the exoteric practices of raja yoga viz. yama, niyama, asana, pranayama.

Bandhas – internal flexions to control the involuntary muscles of the body and release psychic knots and prana.

Basti – internal cleansing technique in which air or water is sucked in through the anus and then evacuated out of the anus again.

Bhagavad Gita – scripture based on the dialogue between Krishna and Arjuna on the subject of yoga.

Bhakti yoga – the yoga of devotion to a personal form of God.

Bhastrika pranayama – a rapid-breathing exercise in which the lungs work like a bellows.

Bhramari pranayama – breathing exercise in which a humming sound is made on exhalation.

Bhrukuti – point between the eyebrows.

Bhujangasana – the serpent pose; a backward-bending posture.

Brahma nada – sound vibration from which all creation emanates, i.e. *om* mantra or cosmic sound.

Chidakasha – the darkness seen behind closed eyes; the abstract, unconscious existence or mind plus self.

Chidakasha vidya – technique of meditation for self-realization.

Chit – mind-stuff.

Chitta – lower mind; memory.

Dhanurasana – bow pose; a backward-bending posture.

Dharana – concentration; continued or exclusive attention to the one object of idea.

Dhauti – hatha yoga technique for internal cleansing.

Dhyana – meditation.

Guru – spiritual guide; dispeller of darkness.

Ha – the first syllable of 'hatha', representing vital energy which flows through pingala (surya) nadi.

Halasana – plough pose; a forward-bending asana.
Ham – the sound vibration of the outgoing breath.
Hatha yoga – the yogic path that is primarily concerned with bodily purification practices which tranquillize the mind and discipline the body, i.e. the balance of ida and pingala nadis.
Hridaya chakra – the heart centre.
Ichha – will; desire fixed or set by the will.
Ida – one of the three main pranic channels in the human body; also known as mental or moon flow.
Ishta devata – desired deity or object of meditation.
Ishta mantra – one's 'desired' or chosen mantra.
Ishwara – God; the Supreme Giver.
Ishwara pranidhana – fixing the mind on the meditation centre.
Jala – the gross element water.
Japa – repetition of a mantra.
Jiva – individual embodied spirit.
Jnana yoga – the yoga of enquiry; the branch of yoga that enables us to know what we are.
Jnanendriyas – sense organs.
Kaki mudra – practices in which the mouth is shaped like a crow's beak and air is steadily inhaled.
Kapalbhati – technique for removing cerebral tension by forceful expulsion of air from the lungs.
Karma yoga – work done with perfect detachment in the pursuit of yoga; exhaustion of abnormal complexes.
Karmendriyas – organs of action.
Khechari mudra – practice in which the tongue is rolled back into the cavity behind the palate and the eyes are focused on the eyebrow centre.
Kumbhaka – retention of breath either inside or outside the body.
Kundalani – the primal energy in man; resides in mooladhara chakra.
Maha mudra – great psychic attitude.
Mala – rosary, usually with 108 beads plus a terminal bead, used for counting during japa.
Manasik japa – mental repetition of a mantra.

Manipura chakra – the psychic centre at the level of the navel, in the spine.

Manomaya kosha – the mental body; one of the five sheaths of human existence.

Mantra – combination of potent sounds which, when repeated, enables the practitioner to reach his goal; usually revealed to rishis in deep meditation.

Matsyasana – fish pose.

Mayurasana – peacock pose.

Mooladhara chakra – the psychic centre between the anus and the genitals at the perineum in males, and at the back of the cervix in females.

Mudra – internal exercise for activating glands; a psychic attitude.

Nabho mudra – 'sky gesture' in which the tongue is rolled back against the roof of the mouth and the eyes are focused on the eyebrow centre.

Nada Brahman – the 'sound cosmos' i.e., the cosmos seen as the manifestation of sound vibrations.

Nada yoga – the science of sound.

Nadi – pranic flow.

Nadi shodhana pranayama – full form of alternate nostril breathing; it purifies the pranic flows.

Nauli – hatha yoga technique for abdominal massaging.

Neti – the hatha yoga technique for nasal cleansing.

Nishkam mantra – mantra repeated without any selfish interest.

Niyamas – observances of conduct or character; one of the eight limbs of raja yoga.

Om – primal sound from which the universe came into existence.

Padmasana – lotus posture.

Paschimottanasana – forward-bending stretch pose.

Patanjali – author of the 'Yoga Sutras' which are the basis of ashtanga yoga.

Pingala – one of the three main pranic channels in the human body; also called surya (sun) nadi.

Pooraka – inhalation of breath and prana.

Prana – the gross manifestation in the physical body of the subtle, universal, cosmic force that gives life to all beings.

Pranayama kosha – the vital body; one of the five sheaths of human existence.

Pranayama – breathing exercises for the expansion of life force in the body.

Pratyahara – withdrawal or control of the senses.

Prithvi – the gross earth element.

Raja yoga – the system of yoga codified by Patanjali; has eight parts viz. yama, niyama, asana, pranayama, pratyahara, dharana, dhyana, samadhi.

Rechaka – exhalation of breath.

Rishi – seer, saint, sage.

Sadhana – spiritual practice.

Sahita pranayama – simple alternate nostril breathing with breath retention.

Sakam mantra – mantra repeated to achieve a particular end e.g. to cure illness.

Samadhi – the culmination of yogic effort in a super-conscious state of self-equilibrium.

Samana – one of the five manifestations of prana within the human body.

Samaveta pranayama – pranayama in which the breath is inhaled and exhaled through both nostrils simultaneously.

Samskaras – accumulated mental tendencies that are the residue of past experiences.

Sannyasin – renunciate.

Sarvangasana – shoulderstand pose.

Satya – truth.

Shalabhasana – locust posture; a backward-bending pose.

Shambhavi mudra – gesture in which the eyes are focused on the eyebrow centre while concentrating on the inner self.

Shashankasana – the moon posture.

Shatkarmas – the six purificatory techniques of hatha yoga viz. neti, dhauti, basti, nauli, trataka, kapalbhati.

Shavasana – the corpse posture.

Sheetali pranayama – a breathing exercise in which the tongue is extended and rolled into a tube through which air is inhaled.

Sheetkari pranayama – breathing exercise in which air is inhaled through clenched teeth, producing a hissing sound.
Shoonya – the void.
Siddha yoni asana – adept's posture, female version.
Siddhasana – adept's posture, male version.
Sirshasana – headstand pose.
So – the sound vibration of the ingoing breath.
Sphatik mani – crystal ball.
Sukh poorvaka pranayama – a simple alternate-nostril breathing exercise.
Sukhasana – pleasant pose.
Sukshma loka – subtle plane.
Sumeru – the principle bead of a mala, offset from the main loop, which must not be crossed during meditation.
Suptavajrasana – sleeping thunderbolt pose.
Sushumna – the chief pranic channel in the human body; located within the spinal cord.
Swadhisthana – the psychic centre at the base of the spine.
Swadhyaya – self-observation on all levels.
Swara yoga – the yogic science of the breath.
Swastika – Hindu sign of the cross; symbol of auspiciousness.
Swastikasana – the auspicious pose.
Tabula rasa – clean slate.
Tapasya – sustained endurance.
Tha – second syllable of 'hatha' representing mental energy which flows through ida (lunar) nadi.
Trataka – gazing at an object for a long period to develop concentration.
Udana – one of the manifestations of prana within the body.
Uddiyana bandha – an important practice in which the stomach is drawn up under the ribs and the abdomen contracted.
Ujjayi pranayama – breathing exercise where the throat is contracted to give a light snoring sound.
Vajrasana – thunderbolt pose.
Varisar dhauti – (shankhaprakshalana) cleansing of the digestive tract by drinking salt water and performing asanas. The water and stool are then evacuated through the anus.

Vasana – desire.

Vastra dhauti – technique for cleansing the stomach by swallowing and removing a specially prepared cloth.

Vatsar dhauti – technique for gulping air into stomach and then belching at one time through the mouth.

Vayu – the gross air element.

Vedas – ancient Indian scriptures.

Vidya – spiritual knowledge; meditation.

Vijnanamaya kosha – the higher mental (intuitive) body; one of the five sheaths of human existence.

Vishuddhi – the psychic centre located at the level of the throat in the spine.

Vyana – one of the five manifestations of prana in the human body.

Yamas – moral abstinences; one of the eight limbs of raja yoga.

Yoga – union of individual and supreme self; the practical means used to attain this union.

Yoga mudra – yogi's posture; a forward-bending pose.

Yoga nidra – psychic sleep; the sleep of the yogis.

Publications

Collections of Satsangs/Discourses

Bhakti Yoga Sagar, Vol. I to VII
Swami Satyananda (1994–2001)
Early Teachings of Swami Satyananda
On the Wings of the Swan, Vol. I to IV
Swami Niranjanananda (1987–1993)
Steps to Yoga
Letters by Swami Satyananda
Taming the Kundalini
Letters by Swami Satyananda
Teachings of Swami Satyananda, Vol. I to VI
Yoga From Shore To Shore
Swami Satyananda's first world tour (1968)
Yoga Sadhana Panorama, Vol. I, II & III
Swami Niranjanananda (1994–97 satsangs given in India, Australia, & Europe)

Yoga Practices

Asana Pranayama Mudra Bandha
Dharana Darshan
Dynamics of Yoga
Kundalini Tantra
Meditations from the Tantras
Moola Bandha, The Master Key
Nawa Yogini Tantra
Practical Yoga Psychology
Prana Pranayama Prana Vidya
Sure Ways to Self-Realization
Surya Namaskara
A Systematic Course in the Ancient Tantric Techniques of Yoga and Kriya
Tattwa Shuddhi: The Tantric Science of Inner Purification
Yoga Education for Children
Yoga Nidra

Health Management

Effects of Yoga on Hypertension
Practices of Yoga for the Digestive System
Yoga and Cardiovascular Management
Yogic Management of Asthma and Diabetes
Yogic Management of Common Diseases

Yoga and Tantra – Texts and Tradition

Four Chapters on Freedom: Commentary on Yoga Sutras of Patanjali
Hatha Yoga Pradipika
Ishavasya Upanishad
Karma Sannyasa
Light on the Guru-Disciple Relationship
Nine Principal Upanishads
Prashnopanishad
Sannyasa Darshan
Siddha Stotra Mala: A Garland of Chants
Sri Vijnana Bhairava Tantra: The Ascent
Swara Yoga: The Tantric Science of Brain Breathing
Yajna: A Comprehensive Survey
Yoga Chudamani Upanishad: Crown Jewel of Yoga
Yoga Darshan: Vision of the Yoga Upanishads

Notes